THE Fitness Response™

21 Steps to 'Model' Your Way To a Fit, FABULOUS BODY!

Richard Kelley, M.D.

SHE Inc. Publishing
an imprint of Morgan James Publishing
NEW YORK

THE **Fitness** Response™

21 Steps to 'Model' Your Way to a Fit, Fabulous Body

Published in New York, New York, by Morgan James Publishing. Morgan James is a trademark of Morgan James, LLC. www.MorganJamesPublishing.com

The Fitness Response, Living the Fitness Response, The Fit Kit, Total Body Muscle Activation, Walking the Edge of Hunger and Physician's Way are trademarks of Physician's Way LLC. The Physician's Way Icon is an exclusive trademark and property of Physician's Way LLC. This book is not intended as a substitute for the medical advice and the supervision of your own primary physician. It is recommended by the author that before undertaking this, or any other program, course of diet, exercise or fitness plan, that you should first consult with your physician.

ISBN 9781614480334 paperback
ISBN 9781614480341 eBook
Library of Congress Control Number: 2011928660

Published by:
SHE Inc. Publishing
an imprint of
MORGAN JAMES PUBLISHING
1225 Franklin Ave. Ste 325
Garden City, NY 11530-1693
Toll Free 800-485-4943
www.MorganJamesPublishing.com

Cover Design by:
Ravi Verma
www.rdezines.com

Interior Design by:
Bonnie Bushman

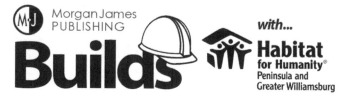

In an effort to support local communities, raise awareness and funds, Morgan James Publishing donates a percentage of all book sales for the life of each book to Habitat for Humanity Peninsula and Greater Williamsburg.

Get involved today! Visit
www.MorganJamesBuilds.com

To my parents, Bill and Pat Kelley, all of my brothers and sisters, and to my wonderful wife, Sherrill: And to my son, Jake: May you dream big and follow your heart where it leads you, knowing that anything you desire is possible and fully within your reach, if you will follow your dreams and dare to pursue them with the passion I know is inside you.

Table of Contents

Introduction

I was startled awake by my pager. Was it 6 a.m. already? Somehow I had managed to doze off at the nurses' station while writing admission orders for the last trauma patient that I would ever see as a general surgery resident at LSU Medical Center in Shreveport, Louisiana.

I had begun my final night of call on the last evening of June 1996, leading into the first day of July, the long-standing nationwide changeover date in hospitals across the country, in which graduating medical students enter teaching hospitals to begin their trial by fire training to become real doctors.

As for me, this last night on call, wrapped up three years of general surgery training, three of the most demanding work years that I have yet to face in my adult life. My particular teaching hospital boasted a Regional Burn Unit and a Level 1 Trauma Center and as such, there seemed to be a non-stop barrage of burn injuries, stabbings, motor vehicle collision injuries, and assaults, all of which fell under the responsibility of the general surgery service. And as usual, it was an all night affair.

It was commonplace as a medical or surgical resident in the early to mid-1990s to still work hospital hours in excess of 100 hours per week. This practice has since changed, as a result of litigation which followed the 1984 hospital death of Libby Zion, a young woman whose demise in a New York hospital under the care of an exhausted and possibly overly stretched resident house staff led to limiting residents to no more than 80-hospital hours of work per week, among other stipulations for oversight.

Nevertheless, as a surgical resident in the 90s, my call responsibility fell to every third night on an ongoing basis. It was understood that you did not leave the hospital, until all of your team's work was complete and you handed responsibility for your surgical service, for the night, over to the oncoming resident on-call.

As opposed to many other occupations, at that time, there was an unwritten understanding that you did not call in sick unless you were ill enough to be admitted to the hospital. <u>On-call</u> meant that you arrived at the hospital around 5 to 6 a.m. for patient rounds, spent your day either in clinic or in the operating room, and after completing evening rounds, you were handed the pagers or beepers from other services that you would cover for the night.

Then, depending on what might be happening in the hospital that evening, you would spend most of the night awake in the emergency department sewing lacerations and dealing with trauma, or in the operating room, operating on individual trauma patients.

Twenty-four hours after you arrived at the hospital, and after being up all night long, it was again time to start morning patient rounds. After completing morning rounds, you would then be off and running to either clinic or the operating room for the new day's work, followed again by afternoon or early evening rounds. This generally meant you were at the hospital, awake and working for at least 36 hours straight.

As I answered that final hospital page from the operator, on the morning of July 1, 1996, it seemed as though a huge weight had suddenly been lifted from my shoulders. The sun was coming up, and I handed over my pager to the oncoming surgical resident. In the blink of an eye, it seemed that an ever-pervasive cloak of responsibility for the ill, battered, broken, and sick had miraculously been lifted.

Suddenly I had a one-year reprieve from the every-third-night call schedule that had dictated every aspect of my life for what had seemed like an eternity. The fourth year in my particular residency program was slated as a lab research year. As such, it was much more relaxed and essentially a vacation from the demands of day-to-day patient care.

It was during this time that I made the realization I had gained about 30 pounds over the course of the three previous years. Though my work demands had become significantly less, I suddenly realized that I was very much out of shape.

I had always been fairly fit and had played sports in high school. I continued to exercise regularly, even during my college years, but this weight gain in my early 30s was something entirely new to me and something I truly had little personal experience dealing with.

To make a long story short, during my research year, I reconnected with the women I would later marry. I did some hospital emergency room work to make some extra money and to stay busy. I was fortunate at this time to have the opportunity to reflect a little on my life up to that point, and I ultimately made the decision not to return to the surgical training program. This decision made a huge change in my life, because the past three years' demands, intensity, and challenges literally shaped me in so many ways.

Ultimately, I determined that becoming a surgeon was simply not the best fit for me. Fortunately, however, the skills that I took from surgical and trauma training, transferred well to a newfound passion for emergency medicine. I liked the variety of patient care in the ER and the excitement of it all. However, in the emergency department, I also began to notice the ramifications and manifestation of poor lifestyle choices that people often make, and I realized that much of what is seen and cared for in that setting is to some degree self-inflicted.

I cared for those with emphysema and COPD (chronic obstructive lung disease) from a lifetime of smoking. I also cared for a 34-year-old heart attack victim who was markedly overweight, smoked, and whose wife "ratted him out" to me about how horrible his dietary habits were. I treated heroine and methamphetamine addicts, chronic alcoholics, and patients who had diabetes and hypertension secondary to their excess weight or obesity.

Along the way, I realized that I needed to get my own physical house in order.

Having seen so much illness and pathology associated with the overindulgence, self-abuse and neglect that are so prevalent in a hospital environment, I knew I did not want to travel down that path.

I also knew I needed to lose weight and become fit again. Fortunately, I not only learned how to do it, but through my own personal and professional experience, I have developed the knowledge, and expertise to teach others how to do it, and it has changed my life forever.

I am writing this book because I know that you too may be looking to change your life. You may think that you have done everything possible to lose weight and improve your health. However, if you are still struggling, there is a distinct possibility that you have not done or tried everything.

Over the past 15 years, I have devoted myself to learning about how the "fittest of the fit" lose weight and change their bodies. If change is what you are seeking, my goal is to hand you the keys and give you the tools to help make it happen once and for all. I have helped many men and women just like you reach the weight-loss and fitness goals that they once believed were simply not possible.

I know that you can do it as well, and I want to help you.

The Decision to Change: Why It Matters

It is no secret that many, many of us are overweight. In fact, more of us are overweight and out of shape than at any other time in history. In my own near half-century on this planet, I have grown from my childhood through a time when being obese seemed a rare exception in our society. Often referred to as a glandular problem, it was just not well understood by the population at large. Fast-forward to where we are today with well over 65% of the adult population either overweight or obese.

Given the enormous numbers that this entails, you or someone close to you may be struggling with this issue and quite possibly have no clue how to change. Sitting to observe people at any public location or event gives an almost certain sense of validity that obesity is a problem almost too large and daunting to solve. Certainly, there appears to be no single, easy solution.

Because being overweight has become so commonplace, I believe that even as physicians who have an eye out for pathology in our patients, the tendency to see excess weight as outside the norm, to some degree has become blunted, because in fact, overweight has become the statistical norm.

I recently saw a new patient who is well over 100 pounds overweight. But because her most recent lab work from her primary doctor "looked fine," she said, "they told me I was healthy."

In fact, the market has readily made great strides to adapt to the new norm. Plus-size clothing stores have opened, furniture makers have responded by increasing chair and sofa sizes with increased durability, restaurants everywhere have ramped up to give patrons the option for all-you-can-eat buffets and all of these changes have become commonplace in a relatively short span of time.

The numbers, in fact, are so great that the obesity epidemic has led to a boom in another industry. The demand for oversized caskets has been on the rise for the last 10 to 15 years. According to an Associated Press release from June 18, 2010, "Indiana casket maker Keith Davis, owner of Goliath Casket, says as Americans get fatter he's trying to accommodate their girth—in death. At 4 feet 4 inches wide…the caskets are the size of a compact car and his business is booming courtesy of the growing obesity epidemic."

This problem is bad, and I suspect it will only get worse. We have reached a point where local city government in some regions of the country, have begun to impose their divine will upon the people. Just recently, the city of San Francisco passed an ordinance prohibiting the inclusion of toys in so-called "happy meals" for kids, following the lead of a similar measure passed months back in Santa Clara County, unless the meals met a specific set of nutrition guidelines.

You may have also heard about New York Mayor Michael Bloomberg's push to encourage the commercial food industry to begin reducing the amount of sodium in a wide array of products. The goal of this would result in a 25% reduction in the nation's salt intake over the next 5 years.

Will these measures be better for our overall health? Possibly they will, some might argue, but where does it end? Do you really want to live in a nation where your right to choose what you eat and how much should be dictated by the government? I certainly do not.

However, the fact remains, that as a nation, we are not eating well. We are not taking care of ourselves and we are getting fat. We are out of shape, and there is no collective solution in sight.

On the other hand, the lens through which we view this issue varies greatly. There are certainly many among us who don't view excess weight as a problem at all. Many men, for example, appear quite confident sporting a sizable beer belly, and culturally we don't seem to give it a second thought.

For others excess weight is a constant companion, feeding one's sense of pain, frustration, dread, and failure.

For the average person on the street, the sight of an overweight or obese individual might elicit thoughts such as "he's too darn heavy" or "she just should not be wearing that outfit, as big as she is."

Because of my background, however, when I see someone who is obviously overweight or obese, I often see something entirely different. I think, "I bet her cholesterol is high," "I wonder if he has sleep apnea," "she's at high risk of developing deep vein thrombosis," "I wonder if she could have diabetes," "I'll bet he's got hypertension," "she is at risk of sudden death," and so on.

You see, if you are overweight you are at risk of developing weight-related illness. How much risk depends on how overweight you are, your genetic blueprint, and whether you have arrived at a point where your excess weight has begun to negatively affect specific physiologic functions. Although there are exceptions, statistically speaking, as your **Body Mass Index** rises, so too does your risk of developing any number of a long list of ailments directly related to excess weight.

* **BMI** (Body Mass Index) is a measure of your weight in kilograms divided by your height (in meters squared). It implies a risk relationship between height and weight. As weight at a certain height increases beyond a particular point, your risk of developing weight-related illness increases, as well.

So, if any of what I am saying has any relevance to where you are now, I have to ask, "Does it matter to you? Does it matter enough to you to actually do something about it? Or, are you content to wait until you develop some health related issue that forces you to address the problem, or are you content to wait until some external regulatory body imposes its will upon you, forcing you to change, or else?"

The fact is that your health is really up to you. It is your responsibility to take care of yourself. You can decide that it's going to be a priority to you and do something to change it, or you may actually lose your health or lose your ability to choose what is right for you.

You can choose to become healthier than you are now. You can choose to eat in a manner that gives vibrancy and nourishment to your body, and you can choose to make moving, a daily priority.

The time to change is right now. The longer that you wait, the longer your health may be at risk. I am not exaggerating or trying to scare you. Many of the patients that I see in my clinic do what I encourage them to do, and they lose weight and become healthier in the process. Sometimes in as little as only a month or two, their lab work improves, blood pressure goes down, and they invariably say that they feel much better.

There are also patients that I see that, for whatever reason, can't seem to motivate themselves to change, despite my prompting and encouragement. I am fearful for them. Their blood pressure is often high. They may not take their medications properly. They often have elevated blood glucose levels and may be prediabetic or already have developed adult onset diabetes. These patients scare me because I can't live in their shoes, and I can't make the necessary changes for them. I am often afraid for them and for the possibility that at some point they might experience a stroke, heart attack, other cataclysmic event, or sudden death.

I know they have the capacity to change their health by making simple, daily changes and if they refuse to do so, their risk of something bad occurring is a distinct possibility. I want to help these people, and I want to help you, as well.

In writing this book, I am going to focus on what I know. I am going to draw from nearly 20 years of medical experience, as well as from my personal fitness knowledge and experience. But I am also going to draw from and focus on the experience and expertise of individuals outside of the field of medicine, the men and women in our society who really understand how to sculpt, change, and manipulate their physical bodies and live the art and science of doing so. These are athletes, fitness competitors, bodybuilders, and dedicated fitness enthusiasts, amateur and professional, male and female alike.

We are living in unprecedented times. We are surrounded by inexpensive, high-calorie, low-nutrient, high-carbohydrate food, which also just happens to taste good. Yet, we continually hear, "Just park your car farther out in the parking lot," "Just get out and do some gardening to burn extra calories," or "Just make sure you walk 'this many steps' per day," or worse, we're told to simply push ourselves away from the table.

It's true; some of these actions and activities may actually be beneficial in adding to your daily calorie expenditure. However, my experience has led me to conclude that without a consistent and organized plan of exercise, coupled with at least a very conscious plan of nutrition, rarely do people make significant and lasting progress when it comes to making changes in the realm of weight loss. A plan instituting only the trite, road-weary recommendations which I mentioned previously, is usually just plain inadequate for someone who happens to live in the calorie-rich food environment where most Americans live.

So if you are open to learning more about individuals who live a dedicated fitness-based lifestyle, I am here to convey that information. I hope to help you understand why many of the concepts and practices that these individuals employ help them change their bodies in a way that may be foreign to the population at large.

These individuals don't tend to follow the traditional, familiar dietary paths. My goal is to help you understand the most effective aspects of what they do day after day, to achieve the results that they achieve and explain why following certain aspects of their path may help you achieve a fitter, healthier body.

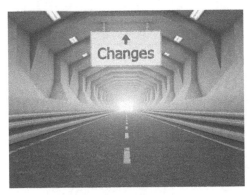

So, if you are struggling with your weight and less than ideal health and you want to learn more, please take the time to keep reading. We all know that words can move us to change. It is my ultimate hope that you will take the words that I have written and do something with them. Today is the day. It is time to make a change. You will not regret doing so. I promise.

Chapter 1

Visualize Change

Do you remember when you were a kid? Anything was possible. You may have made a Christmas list the length of your arm and thought it would all show up on Christmas Eve or Christmas morning.

When you played with your friends, you imagined that you were a gold medal winner in the Olympics, or you were going to become Miss America, or you would drive a racecar one day. Or maybe you were going to become president of the United States. Regardless of how your vision was unique to you, you believed attaining it was something you were going to do, some day.

The blind, optimistic hopes and dreams of youth have no boundaries. However, we all know that as time passes and we grow older with each year, the sense of what we believe we can accomplish can and often does become muffled and stagnant. Certainly our hopes and dreams change as we grow and mature along the way, but something else happens, as well.

We get blindsided by a flippant comment from a teacher or a classmate when we read out loud in class. A coach says he has a basset hound than runs faster than you. Maybe you overhear someone in school make an uncaring remark about your facial features.

Regardless of our youthful hopes, dreams, and ambitions, it is not uncommon for us to lose our self-esteem and confidence as the years, acquaintances, and circumstances of life proceed to deliver a psychological beating. If you've gained excess weight over the years, this can translate into an added sense of self-defeat, over which you might feel you have little control. You may feel you've reached a point where "It just is what it is," and there is nothing more that you can do to change it.

We all feel powerless at times, whether the issue is the inability to advance at a job, difficulty communicating with a spouse or coworker, or knowing that there is a cap on your income. However, when we stand back and look clearly at the circumstances, usually we can do something to alter or improve a given scenario.

You can change jobs, decide to listen more intently to your spouse, or increase your education with the goal of boosting your income. But where your weight and physical body are concerned, you may feel that you have tried everything. Maybe you have spent your entire life dieting, only to have fleeting and periodic success followed by the return of your lost weight, plus more, along with feelings of frustration and defeat.

If this has been your struggle, please take heart. It is often possible to find an answer if you can allow yourself to stand back and take a look in another direction.

For so many of us, the decision to lose weight is tied to the only word we know, diet. It's all about the food and what you can't eat and how little you can eat. It's about starvation and deprivation. It is so painful and discouraging, but it is the only thing we know to do.

Dieting may be the only thing you know how to do, but it is rarely the road to sustained weight loss. There is another way however, a better way, and one that leads to more sustainable weight control, however, you must go back to that place when you were a kid, when anything was possible. In reality, anything you want bad enough is possible.

Just as there is a template for becoming an accountant, a doctor, a lawyer, a gymnast, a musician, an oceanographer, etc., there is a template for you to develop a better body.

For any goal that you want to achieve in life, there are coaches. There is training and schooling, formal or informal, but the information is there. If you want to learn anything at all, there has never been a time in history where the information was more accessible than it is right now. And where there is information, there is usually someone around whose specialty is teaching that information. You just have to decide what it is you want to learn and start looking.

As I said, there is a template for losing weight and changing your body. And there are coaches, teachers, trainers and individuals who have the information and expertise to teach you how.

If you are not currently happy with where you are, I want to encourage you to begin to **visualize** what the best physical version of *you* looks like. Look in the mirror. What would you change? Do you wish you had a leaner midsection? Do you have more flab on your arms than you want? How about your backside? Do you want less than what you have now?

We are all different, we have different features that we may not be happy with, but in general, I believe for many of us there is a healthier, more ideal physical body that we can visualize. There is nothing wrong with imagining a better version of you than you currently see in the mirror. There is nothing wrong with wanting to look better. Often what we see in the mirror is a direct reflection of someone who is not truly caring for themselves and not treating themselves well.

I want you to begin to picture in your mind's eye how you will look on your best day. Maybe you're wearing an outfit that you never thought you could wear. Maybe you're out jogging on the local running trail, lean, fit, and toned, your sweat-glistened skin highlighting a physique with muscle definition, without excess fat. Maybe you are attending a summer party wearing a sundress that shows off your arms and shoulders, whereas before you would never have been caught dead in an outfit without sleeves.

Get this picture in your head. **Visualize the change.** Define what it looks like.

Now let's reinforce it.

Chapter 2

Find Your Model of Success

Assume that you wanted to learn to paint, how would you start? Maybe your first step would be a drive to the craft store to buy some paints, an easel and a canvas. Would you know what kind of paint to purchase? Oil, watercolor, acrylic? Would you know what kind of brushes you needed?

You could certainly "wing-it" and pick up all of the items you think that you need, head home with a plan to have a go at it, and set up your own spontaneous, improvisational studio in the garage. On your first try, you might find that you are a natural born artist and that your first painting is destined to become a cherished and valuable work of art.

We've all heard stories of this type of thing happening and somewhere out in the world there is surely a prodigy waiting to discover that he or she has this very skill. On the other hand, most of us are not prodigy painters and possibly not prodigy anything, but we all have the ability to learn, and the ability to learn is one of life's most underappreciated gifts.

A more reliable course of action on your quest to become a great painter might be to sign up for a class at your local community college that teaches basic painting skills. You might be surprised to learn that they offer courses in freehand drawing, watercolor, oil, and acrylic painting. You might also find someone who specializes in and teaches the painting style of period-specific works of art such as from the early Renaissance period.

You would also likely be able to find similar classes and expertise in photography, woodworking, piano, effective communication with the opposite sex, quilt making, macramé, Spanish or other languages, psychology, finance, astrology, and more.

Within each of these arts or disciplines, you would most certainly find individuals who were masters at teaching their specialty or craft, as well.

If your goal is to lose weight and to increase your level of fitness, you undoubtedly will find many competent trainers, fitness enthusiasts, nutritionists, and amateur or professional fitness competitors or bodybuilders who have the tools, background, and experience to guide you on a quest to a fitter, leaner body.

Any number of these individuals might also reflect a physical representation and body that you might consider desirable to model. Can you model someone else's physique? Of course you can. Just as you can learn any art or skill that can be taught by someone who has achieved competence in a particular area, you can also find someone who has the general physical characteristics and body type that you desire and can often follow the same or a similar path to a similar outcome.

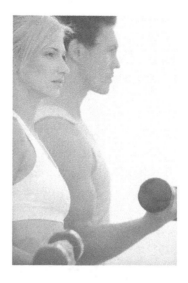

Competitors in the world of bodybuilding have done this forever and if you have ever witnessed a bodybuilding competition, live or otherwise, you may have noted that it is very difficult for the casual, untrained observer to differentiate the sometimes subtle differences between the physiques of various competitors. In fact, if it were not for differences in height and overall weight of these competitors, you might note the general physical characteristics of these individuals to be quite similar.

Why such a close physical resemblance? The answer is modeling. These individuals, though their training methods may vary to a greater or lesser degree, by and large focus on stimulating the muscles of their bodies in a way that produces predictable results which they hope will be found favorable with the judges. Because the most competitive members of the bodybuilding community have a vision of the physical attributes that win bodybuilding competitions, collectively, they are able to reproduce the physical appearance that we all recognize and associate with the practitioners of this particular sport.

Images are powerful. What you focus upon can become reality. A myriad of books and magazines on the market today highlight both men and women who have achieved strong, healthy, powerful physical bodies through hard work and dedication towards a goal.

Monica Brant, champion fitness competitor, fitness cover model, and winner of the 1998 Fitness Olympia, reportedly began lifting weights in 1991, after being inspired by a photo of 1990 Fitness USA Champion, Marla Duncan, in a national fitness magazine.

Possessing one of the most proportionate and classically symmetrical physiques in bodybuilding, Frank Zane, reportedly was 14 years old when he walked into his high school math class and spotted a muscle building magazine in the wastebasket. Studying the magazine, he soon started training at the local Wilkes-Barre YMCA weight room. Training with weights for over 50 years, he has won all of the highest titles in bodybuilding, including defeating Arnold Schwarzenegger for Mr. Universe.

So you certainly can find one or more persons of similar height and body structure who have achieved a specific physical transformation and model their success, by learning the path that they took to reach their goal.

Some may argue that this is not possible or that somehow there is something wrong with trying to emulate the physical attributes of another person. In fact, when it comes to altering one's appearance with cosmetic surgery to look like a celebrity or some completely different individual than oneself and abandoning one's own identity, I would have to agree that this may not, in fact, be healthy.

On the other hand, modeling optimal fitness and the development of a lean, toned, healthy physical body, I believe is a worthwhile goal. I have been in position to observe over and over again the normalization of previously abnormal lab work and blood pressure and even the resolution of adult onset diabetes when people make the decision to take control of their health and fitness, through optimal diet and exercise.

Sure, you could model your neighbor, who lost 15 pounds by eating nothing but pea soup for a month. Or you could do what your sister-in-law did, following a stringent 500-calorie-per-day diet, while receiving hormone injections or you could ask your co-worker, who refers to herself as "a lifetime dieter," what she believes your best route to success may be.

In fact, when I ask new patients, "What brought you in to see me today?" they often respond by saying something like, "My sister in Florida is doing a diet 'just like this' and has lost 20 pounds!" I quickly make it very clear to these patients that the process I teach is based in fitness first, and that they will not simply be placed on "just some diet."

This is where, I believe, we have collectively steered off course. We have reached a place where the <u>majority</u> of adult Americans are now overweight or possibly obese, and yet many of us are asking our friends, family, peers and coworkers, who are often struggling with the same issues, to give us their advice or solution to the problem.

Or we may buy into some commercial dietary approach that has been around for some years, but which breeds dependency on a particular system of calorie counting, brand-specific "diet foods," or other means of quantization of food intake, without teaching an understanding of how food really affects metabolism.

I am adamant in my belief that a dietary approach that excludes fitness as a foundation of good health is generally destined for limited or marginal results, at best, for the long haul.

So having said this, if your goal is to lose weight, improve your body, and increase your fitness, I would encourage you to **find someone whose physical body you would like to emulate: find someone to model**. You don't have to choose someone, necessarily in the fitness or bodybuilding world. You may know someone who lives in your own neighborhood that has the physical attributes that you want to mirror. Perhaps you will, however, find your ideal model in the pages of a fitness magazine or even someone at your local gym.

Wherever you find the person or persons you wish to model, then find out as much about that person as you possibly can. What do they eat? What kinds of exercise do they do? Do they focus on walking, yoga, or Pilates? Do they swim, play tennis, or engage in regular weight-training or resistance exercise? Where do they exercise? How many days do they exercise? Do they follow a specific nutrition plan? Do they adhere to some particular training theory? Are they trying to just not gain weight, or are they trying to build muscle while also decreasing their overall body fat?

If you can speak with your ideal role model personally, you might be surprised to find this person to be very open and generous with their time and information. Often, those who have achieved success in any area are happy that others notice and recognize the success they have a won through hard work and effort. They may be very happy to share both their time and philosophy with an interested party.

My goal is to encourage you to find someone who is living a healthy, fitness-based lifestyle and has some of the physical attributes that you would like to emulate and find out how this person achieved those results. Positive, successful role models are everywhere. You just have to determine what you want to achieve and look for the person or persons who can guide you along a similar path.

Chapter 3

Get Clear about Your Goals

I often see men and women in my clinic who are in their 30s, 40s, 50s and beyond who tell me they would like to reach a weight they were at in their early adulthood. However, many of these patients add, "But I know that's just not realistic at my age."

Having recently read <u>Live Young Forever</u>, written by then-95-year-old health and fitness legend, Jack Lalanne, I realized just how limited our thinking can be, especially when it comes to what is possible with the human body. In fact, there is a picture of Jack Lalanne in his latest book, taken in 1994 at age 80. The caption below says, "I felt in top form at the age of 80, and I could still perform hundreds of pushups. I felt no different than I had at 25, a true testament to sensible exercise and nutrition. But the waistline was now 27 ½ inches—up by a half an inch. Ooops!"

This book is a real eye opener. Jack Lalanne was a true testament to what is possible when someone lives a life that is focused on maintaining optimal health and fitness. Sadly, we lost Jack Lalanne early in 2011. He was a great inspiration to me and to so many others who watched him engage in feats of strength, endurance, and seemingly superhuman acts to mark so many of his landmark birthdays throughout his life. I feel blessed to have lived during this time in history and to have had in our midst a role model such as Mr. Lalanne, who spent his entire life preaching, teaching, and walking his talk.

So what about you? What do you really want to accomplish? Do you want to drop 50 pounds, improve your cholesterol, and decrease your reliance on blood pressure or diabetes medications? Do you want to become more aerobically fit? Do you want to decrease your body-fat percentage while also building some lean muscle and adding more definition and tone to your physique?

We are all different in this regard and have different goals and ideas about what our best body looks like. Certainly some of the patients that I see just want to be "skinny." They want to reach a weight at which they are happy, without gaining muscle or increasing muscle definition. In general, I see this goal much more often in my female patient population, but the trend is changing somewhat.

I am seeing more and more people, both men and women, who want a change in their physical body that reflects an increase in muscle tone, muscle definition, and in some cases, an increase in overall muscle mass. With rare exceptions, most of these individuals voice that they would also like to become more fit and have more energy with which to pursue their lives.

This statement is strictly based on my own personal contact and experience with the patients that I see in my weight-management practice. However, it is also influenced by the fact that I've seen and cared for thousands of patients over close to 20 years in the medical field and have spent a lot of time asking these people about their goals for their health.

The bottom line is this. If you want to change your body, improve it, and transform it, you need to get clear about what it is that you want to accomplish. The person who just wants to be skinny is often on a different path than the person who wishes to become lean, more muscularly defined, and fit.

The goals which are consistent with these two outcomes will usually be different, as well. In my experience, many people who just want to be skinny tend to spend their lives dieting. The path to skinny is often fraught with discomfort, constant hunger and caloric deprivation. For the most part, I am neither a fan nor advocate of this path, for it typically ignores fitness as a component of overall health.

My experience informs me that many on this path may be less concerned with improving their overall health than with simply being thin. Can you be thin or skinny and be healthy too? Of course you can. However, I have noticed over the years that a subset of this particular group will have little interest in exercise and fitness and tend to approach the path to skinny purely by daily calorie deprivation, if not some form of intentional starvation.

If it is your goal to simply be skinny, I am not your best source of information. However, if your focus is to become more fit and healthier in the process, I am happy to guide you in that direction.

Regardless of what you wish to achieve, whether your goal is simply a weight you've longed to reach or more specifically, a defined physical appearance with specific body measurements, the first step is getting clear on your target and **setting clearly defined goals** to achieve your outcome:

- Do you want to spend your life dieting or are you committed to learning how to eat better and in a manner that supports your fitness and exercise efforts?

- Do you want to lose weight for an upcoming wedding or reunion or do you plan to change your lifestyle to one consistent with the maintenance of your long-term health and fitness?

- Will exercise be something you do only on days that you feel up to it or will it become something you do on a daily basis?

These are all valid questions that you need to ask yourself and get clear about the answers. If you know what it is that you really wish to accomplish, then you can set clearly defined goals about how to proceed.

Do you need a coach, a trainer, or a nutritionist to help you define your path to reaching these goals? Only you can answer that. However, enlisting someone who knows how to guide you along the path to achieving physical change is often helpful and can save you time.

As you continue reading, I am going to lay out the nuts and bolts of what I believe can help you change your body, specifically if you are seeking to lose excess weight and body fat, increase your level of fitness, and possibly increase your muscle definition and tone.

If your overall goals are consistent with any of these things, then by all means read on.

Chapter 4

The Fitness Response™

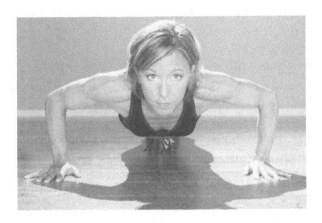

The Fitness Response is a process, which is similar in some regards to a **call and response**, such as that found as a basic element of musical form. In music we often see a set pattern, such as a verse or verses followed by the chorus.

As it pertains to weight loss, optimizing one's level of fitness or completely transforming the physique, those who capitalize on The Fitness Response, do so because they give themselves no other option. Just as in music, a verse is followed by the chorus, such it is with The Fitness Response, a consistent, planned exercise or workout is followed by very specific, often predetermined dietary choices.

Those who are successful in reaching a physical goal that burns in their mind's eye leave little room for error. They embark on a

planned physical activity (the call) on a specific day of the week, and they often follow that exercise with very specific dietary choices **(the response)**. There is no cheesecake reward at the end of their day, just because they exercised.

In the most basic sense, success with The Fitness Response is closely tied to the manifestation of two words: *consistency* and *honesty*. Those who are *honest* with themselves about whether they are exercising and **honest** about what that they are eating, ultimately have more clarity than those who are less than honest with themselves about what they are doing.

Consistency in both diet and exercise is a central key to success, where fitness and weight-loss are concerned, and is the foundation upon which The Fitness Response is based.

This may sound somewhat esoteric; however, you can visualize the day-to-day application of The Fitness Response by looking at how someone in the bodybuilding world might approach two days of a particular week.

Let's take, for theoretical example, Sara, an amateur bodybuilder who has the goal of competing in her first stage competition within the year. In the course of a typical week, Sara might plan to hit the gym six out of seven days, with one day off for rest. Let's say that Day #1 is Monday, and she has decided in advance that Monday is bicep and triceps day and gym time starts at 6 a.m. sharp.

Using The Fitness Response, Sara knows that there is only one goal upon which she needs to focus this morning. Sara chooses to precede this workout by first drinking a protein shake with a very specific target amount of protein for her body weight and with the understanding that today is a day completely focused on stimulating her triceps and bicep muscles through resistance training.

Upon arrival to the gym, Sara proceeds to the free-weight area and goes through a well thought-out resistance training routine in which both the muscles of the biceps and triceps are targeted through a specific number of repetitions, a predetermined approach as to how much weight will be used for each exercise and each given muscle group, as well as how much time she will spend at the gym.

After completion of this workout, Sara then goes home and **responds** to her now completed workout by consuming a six egg-white omelet with steamed spinach, one slice of whole wheat toast, and 8 ounces of water.

The following day is Tuesday. Tuesday just happens to be a straight aerobic or cardiovascular day for Sara. Again, gym time is planned for 6 a.m. However, today the plan is to go to the gym without taking in any calories or nutrition before some light stretching and then running on the treadmill for 45 minutes. Today, Sara is planning to encourage her body to meet its energy needs (burn calories) during the treadmill run by dipping into stored body-fat.

After hitting a specific target heart rate or a specific pace on the treadmill and completing 45 minutes, pausing only to hydrate with water, Sara ends her workout. She heads back home for a post-workout meal, before showering and heading off to work. The ride back to Sara's house takes about 30 minutes; so she is counting on burning some extra calories during the ride home, as her body returns to its pre-workout metabolic state.

Upon arrival home, Sara prepares her post-workout meal. Today is much the same as yesterday, a six egg-white omelet with steamed spinach, but today, she eats no toast with the meal. Today the strategy is to back off of any starchy carbohydrate during the first meal or two of the day. The strategic plan, again, being to 'encourage the body' to continue its trend to burn a few more fat-stored calories over the ensuing hour, by strategically eliminating any 'starchy' forms of carbohydrate (more on this later) during this particular first meal of the day.

The remainder of each of these two days is very predictable for Sara, as well. Mid-morning she has a protein shake and ½ banana; lunch consists of grilled tilapia, a small sweet potato with a squeeze of lemon, and a side of steamed broccoli. Mid-afternoon, she has another whey protein shake with ½ cup of blueberries. For dinner, she eats a medium-size grilled chicken breast, large bowl of steamed spinach, and ½ cup of brown rice. Before bedtime, to give her body something with which it can repair and strengthen muscle during the night's sleep, she consumes a cup of low-fat cottage cheese.

You can view the plan for the remainder of her week in her journal, as follows:

Wednesday: Chest and Shoulder training and 20 minutes of cardio on treadmill

Thursday: 45 minutes of cardio on the treadmill

Friday: Back and abdominal muscles plus 20 minutes cardio on treadmill

Saturday: 20 minutes of cardio on treadmill, followed by leg training

Sunday: Off

Sunday evening, Sara will plan the next week's workout schedule. She may change the order of how various muscle groups are targeted with resistance exercise, along with altering how much aerobic/cardiovascular exercise, or both will be included. Regardless, her diet still consists of a well-thought out stream of calories with specific macronutrient (protein, carbohydrate, fat) content, designed to complement and *respond* to each day's particular exercise demand and training routine for each muscle group.

This is the essence of The Fitness Response: A planned, predetermined course of exercise is embarked upon (**the call**) and it is followed immediately thereafter and throughout the day by specific, predetermined dietary choices (**the response**) designed to elicit a desired, long-term physical outcome.

If you have ever wondered why many athletes and professional fitness competitors look the way they do, it is because they live like most other people don't. Their exercise is planned. Their diet is planned, and those who are the best at what they do rarely deviate. Are they more disciplined than other people? Yes, often they are. On the other hand, they are not superhuman, and their actions, as I've said, can be modeled. These individuals have simply decided what it is that they want their physical body to reflect, and they go about doing time-tested exercise, followed by **specific dietary responses**, to get where they want to go.

Are Sara's friends envious of the way she looks? Many of them are. Do they understand why she has the body that she has? Possibly some of them do. However, there are inevitably those who say, "She's just genetically gifted, because I exercise too and my arms will never look that good." Do Sara's friends see that she approaches her training and her diet in a way that is dramatically different from what they do? Likely, they do not. They might see glimpses here and there. They may know that if they meet her for lunch, she seems to always order a salad topped with grilled salmon and always uses a squeeze of lemon as her salad dressing.

They may also dismiss her as being a bit elusive, because she seems to turn down most offers to go out at night for Mexican food and margaritas. If she does go out, they notice that she never surpasses the one, or maximum of two glasses of wine that she nurses during the evening. Despite the appetizers ordered, she will wait to eat anything until her grilled chicken and veggies arrive with her fajita plate, even to the extent of avoiding a single tortilla from the chip basket, from which her friends cannot keep their hands away.

Do they like Sara? Yes, they do, but some may not understand her very well, or for that matter, what seems to motivate the lifestyle she lives. They are intrigued that she can maintain her weight and appears so fit, while some of them struggle constantly.

Some of Sara's friends may even believe that they exercise just as much as she does, but they feel somehow cheated that they can't replicate her results. Deep down, they may actually believe that Sara just has more time to exercise or less responsibility than they themselves do. Somehow, they believe that for Sara, things must just come a little easier.

In reality, they are wrong; and deep down, they know this too. Because each of Sara's friends knows that their only form of exercise is taking the dog out for a walk two or three times each week. They tell themselves, "I already do so much walking at my job each day and that counts as my exercise."

On the rare occasion that they actually do make it to the gym, to jog or walk on the treadmill or use the elliptical trainer, they have already made the mental negotiation that <u>because</u> they are doing this, they surely have earned the fettuccine alfredo, with half a bottle of wine followed by a slice of "the best cheesecake you ever put in your mouth," which they know at this very moment will be their hard-earned reward.

Sara's friends may <u>say</u> that they want to lose weight, but their actions fail to match up with their words in any meaningful or strategic way. Most of them believe they have tried every diet under the sun, and they have been successful for short periods of time, only to gain their weight back. They often skip breakfast or may have a bagel to start their day and complain that they are constantly hungry. Ironically, Sara knows exactly what she is going to eat on almost any given day, and she is less driven toward food <u>by hunger</u>, than are her friends.

As you can see, there is a great divide, a big disconnect between how Sara lives in comparison with her friends. Is Sara just gifted? Does Sara have some secret that is known only to her? No. What Sara does have is a vision of what she wants her body to look like, and she enacts a plan each and every day that is congruent with the attainment of her vision.

Now, I must admit that this example may possibly be offensive to some who read it and my intent is not to offend or anger you. Sara is a fictitious figure, and her example is strictly my distillation of what I know to be a common approach to the process of physical transformation.

However, I do want to impress upon you that often those individuals who are consistently successful in their efforts to lose weight and keep that weight off are usually doing things in a consistent manner that may fall outside the day-to-day activities and dietary norms of their peers.

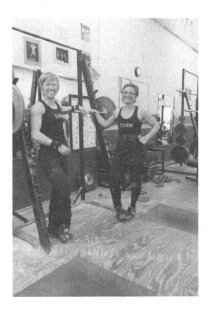

Pattie Farley and Amalia Litras at Hyde Park Gym in Austin, Texas

Pattie and Amalia

Living in Austin, Texas, I have had the good fortune to meet and collaborate with many fitness minded individuals, who bear out, to a great degree, the concept of The Fitness Response.

Pattie Farley and Amalia Litras are two such individuals with whom I have had the pleasure of working with in the past and whose day-to-day lifestyles validate much of what I teach and encourage at my clinic, Physician's Way Healthy Weight Loss. I also want to emphasize that they are not patients of mine, nor are they connected in any way to my practice.

Pattie and Amalia are co-owners of GrassIron, a fitness and personal training organization here in Austin, where they teach and train individuals who have a wide variety of goals, from simply losing weight, to training for a variety of sport-specific strength, speed, or endurance events. They have helped many individuals, male and female, young and old alike, reach personal goals and overcome fitness obstacles and limiting beliefs about what is physically possible.

Not only do they teach and train others to excel, Pattie and Amalia are a testament to living a lifestyle that is grounded in fitness, and as I alluded to previously, they exemplify day-to-day habits which likely set them apart from many other women of similar age, and particularly from those who approach weight loss from a diet-only strategy.

I had the opportunity to ask them a few questions and get their thoughts regarding how they each approach their own training and nutrition, as well as asking them about some of the struggles that they see their clients facing. This is what they had to say:

Question: How do you view yourselves, in terms of your pursuits? Meaning, are you an amateur or professional fitness athlete, bodybuilder, power-lifter, or fitness coach, or something else entirely?

Amalia: Although I am nearly 40 years of age, I am still able to compete in Olympic-style weightlifting on a national level. So for now, I still train as a competitive athlete.

Pattie: I competed in amateur natural bodybuilding from 2001 to 2005. I have competed in power lifting from 2001 to the present and also train for, but do not currently compete in, Olympic-style weightlifting. I have also competed in cycling and running, placing in numerous events. I identify as a strength and conditioning specialist (CSCS) and I am certified through NSCA. I have been a personal trainer for over eight years and have coached sedentary individuals from ages 14 to 75 to become competitive athletes.

Question: How <u>planned</u> is your diet and nutrition? Do you eat randomly during day, but with a fitness-oriented mindfulness, or do you eat in a specific, planned manner each day (i.e., pack a cooler or eat specific foods on a daily basis or at specific restaurants)? Do you have specific calorie, protein, carbohydrate, and fat targets that you aim for?

Amalia: Although I track macronutrients and calories *nearly* every day (I use the app MyFitnessPal), I do not pack a cooler each morning. I eat a healthy breakfast before leaving the house (usually oatmeal, protein powder, and fruit), rely on protein drink or bar for a snack while I'm at work or the gym, and eat lunch and dinner at home. As a competition draws near, I am even more conscientious of food intake so that "making weight" does not become an issue.

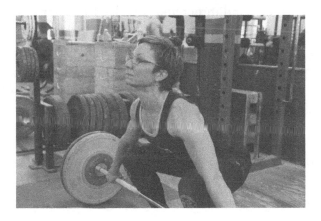

Amalia Litras performing a power lift at Hyde Park Gym

Pattie: My diet and nutrition is extremely planned when it comes to content, but timing is a bit more flexible. I set calories (and macronutrients) based on my current goals, (i.e., fat loss, weight loss, muscle gain, or maintenance) and this varies throughout the year, whether I have a competition and need to make a weight class or just have a body composition goal in mind. I also monitor calories when trying to maintain my body weight or I will surely gain more fat than I prefer to carry! I prepare most of my meals for the week on Sunday or make sure that I have plenty of lean protein and veggies in the fridge that are ready to be cooked on the indoor grill at a moments notice. You will not find much or any junk in my fridge or pantry. I just don't keep it in the house. My will power is not great if it's in my reach. So I just don't keep it around. I do allow myself some guilty pleasures, but moderation is the key, as with anything.

I use an app like MyFitnessPal or Fitday to track my nutrition and activity level. The only time I do not use this method is when on vacation and some occasional weekend trips. **I am in general always mindful of my nutrition.**

My days are unpredictable and busy; so I make sure I start with a good breakfast (i.e., egg whites and turkey bacon and fruit, or oatmeal and protein powder) and throughout the day I may eat protein bars or drink protein shakes. I generally get home for lunch and eat something containing a lean protein and complex carbohydrate (i.e., chicken breast and sweet potato, and something green!). Dinner is more of the same with more veggies. I often like a snack before bed with Greek yogurt, protein powder, and berries. I do love wine; so a glass or two of that is figured in somewhere, unless I really have to cut calories!

Question: How many days each week do you each engage in some form of structured, specific exercise? (aerobic exercise, resistance training, flexibility exercise, etc.)

Amalia: I engage in some form of exercise every single day, even if it's only a walk. I train for my sport (weightlifting) 4–5 times a week, commute by bike 30 miles a week (depending on the season), and walk daily.

Pattie: 6–7 days per week. I lift 4–5 days per week, walk 30–60 minutes every day, bike as a form of commuting a few times per week, and occasionally throw in some 30–45 minute elliptical sessions as needed, if trying to cut weight and for my own sanity! (It feels good to sweat!)

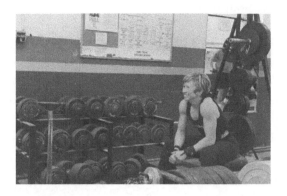

Pattie Farley taking a break between sets at Hyde Park Gym

Question: Do either of you supplement with non-whole food products, such as protein shakes or protein or energy bars, to meet your fitness and dietary needs and goals?

Amalia: Although I recognize the importance of eating whole foods whenever possible, I do supplement with either a protein bar or drink during the day.

Pattie: Yes, we love Perfect Foods Bars and an occasional Builder Bar. These are meal replacements and I treat them as such or eat half as a snack. We drink RTD protein drinks such as Muscle Milk Light or Pure Pro's. These help with hunger cravings and get my protein up to meet my daily goals.

Question: Do either of you view your fitness as a temporary part of your life, meaning maybe it's something you feel is necessary while you're younger, but maybe you'll give yourself a break down the road. Or the opposite, do you view fitness as something you believe you will always pursue?

Amalia: I believe that I will always prioritize fitness in my life. I love a physical challenge. I love feeling strong and self-sufficient. I cannot imagine a life without physical activity.

Pattie: There is nothing temporary about fitness. I hope I am always physically and mentally able to pursue new goals pertaining to fitness. My training was all over the place when I was a bit younger (marathon running to power lifting), and I am more focused on power or speed movements now while I can still get a bit faster. At age 40, that window will start to close over the next few years; so perhaps I will go back to more endurance-based sports later in life. Strength training is a constant, and watching my mother literally shrink and crumble from osteoporosis in front of my very eyes will hopefully serve as a reminder of this: "Use it or lose it." I firmly believe that our bodies are meant to move and that sweat is the best therapy around; so while I may not always compete, I am sure I will still stay very active, as long as I am able.

Question: What do you perceive to be your most prized benefits of living a fitness-based lifestyle? This could be the aesthetics of being fit, some metabolic benefit, the way you feel in general, or something entirely different.

Amalia: Being self-sufficient and being able to overcome obstacles on my own. I had been training a 69-year old woman for nearly 5 years when she came into the gym on a Monday morning with the following announcement:

> "This weekend when I was cutting the grass, I got something caught under the mower. I didn't want to go inside to get my husband, so I got into my dead lift stance, set my back, and tipped it on its side—all by myself! I didn't get hurt! I was so proud of myself that I had to stop what I was doing, go inside, go online, and see how much it weighed!" At that moment I thought, "That's it. That's exactly why we do this." (And by "we," I do mean the both of us!)

Pattie: A general sense of well-being is the biggest benefit in my opinion. Setting and reaching goals is rewarding, and breaking through barriers is rewarding both physically and mentally. The aesthetics of being fit are for sure a great benefit, but that is just a bonus. I feel most in control of all things in my life when my workouts are getting done and my nutrition is on track.

I look back at climbing a hill on my bike or lifting a heavy weight, and I know that I can accomplish anything that set out to accomplish. I know that I can get through any adversity.

It is important to enjoy the journey to the destination because it is not just about the end but all the little milestones along the way.

Question: What are the top struggles your clients tell you they face?

Amalia: Being able to *consistently* make healthy food choices. It's difficult to make a change initially, and then it's difficult to maintain those healthy habits when the novelty wears off.

Pattie: Portion control is probably at the top of the list, followed by making healthy food choices, especially at the office or while traveling, consistency in food logging (they only want to log it when they "have a good eating day"), and they struggle to get extra workouts in even if it's walking.

Question: What are the biggest obstacles you believe most people face when starting a program to get fit or lose weight?

Amalia: In my experience, one of the biggest obstacles is not knowing how or where to begin. The amount of information available online is overwhelming (and contradictory). The fear of failure is also an enormous obstacle when deciding to invest time and money in your health and well-being. We've all bought fitness equipment that we barely use and memberships to a gym that we rarely visit.

Pattie: One of the biggest obstacles seems to be time commitment. No one "has time" but we all make time when it becomes important enough. I think people know that they have to commit for life and that seems daunting, so it is easier to just put it off. The approach in my opinion should be the opposite: better get started now.

There is always some birthday or some vacation planned or some big project at the office, or something that will sabotage their goals. There will always be those things; so it's best to just start the lifestyle change and learn to balance these things as they come.

Final Question: What is the main philosophy at GrassIron that you teach?

Pattie and Amalia: We really encourage our folks to use positive statements to set specific, *performance-based goals* (not outcome-based goals) with a realistic end date. For example: "I want to set a personal record during my next fun run" is a much better goal than "I want to finish in the top 25% of my age group during the next fun run." It is important to set goals over which one has the most control possible.

It is very clear that Pattie and Amalia take their fitness seriously, as well as the fitness of their clients. They understand what it takes to arrive at that place, where one has a greater deal of control over weight, fitness, and wellbeing, and how to live there indefinitely, by doing certain specific things day-in and day-out, from the standpoint of optimal nutrition and exercise.

Do you have to follow a bodybuilding regimen to create change or lose excess weight? Not necessarily, but whatever path to fitness you choose usually requires a high level of both **honesty** and **consistency**. I have a patient that I see in our clinic who lost over 100 pounds this past year, simply by walking every day and eating in a very specific manner. Is she using **The Fitness Response**? Absolutely she is.

This patient continues to walk every day, despite the fact that on some days she may not feel like doing it. She makes it a point to eat 5 to 6 times during each day, and she doesn't deviate much. She has a plan and a very specific goal for where it is that she is going. I have no doubt she will reach her ultimate goal because her efforts are honest, consistent, and congruent with the outcome she is seeking. If she happens to have an off week, I never hear her make excuses. She just resets her plan of action and gets back on course. Her thoughts and actions are congruent with the lighter, healthier body that she can see in her mind's eye.

I want you to realize, that a great body, one that is fit, lean, strong and toned, is <u>earned</u>. It is no accident when certain individuals are able to maintain a high level of fitness through their 40s, 50s, up to 80 and beyond. These individuals are high achievers, where their health and body are concerned. Growing older gracefully with strength and dignity is a priority to them and it should become one for you, as well.

The essence of **The Fitness Response** is simple. It is nothing more than a pattern of **call and response**. It is specific, daily exercise followed by specific, well-planned dietary choices on a consistent and ongoing basis, nothing more. Once you've decided you are truly ready to change, you can implement the Fitness Response to help you get where you want to go, with the peace of mind that your consistency will carry you to your ultimate goal. The first step is figuring out what it is you wish to achieve. In doing so, you will be well on your way to changing your body and developing the tools and habits necessary to maintain positive and lasting change, for as long as you wish.

Chapter 5

Light the Morning Fire

Many of the patients that come to see me for help losing weight complain that they are constantly hungry; in fact, they will tell me that by the time the evening rolls around, they are ravenous.

When we begin to discuss their usual dietary habits, it often becomes very clear to me just why they feel the way that they do. These patients are almost always sincere and well-meaning when they tell me, "I feel like I eat really healthy."

If weight-loss is one of your goals or if you want to create an optimal physiology, one that will help you lose weight, you must take what I'm about to say to heart. If you ignore my next statement, you are likely to continue to struggle in your efforts to progress. So here it is.

When you go to bed at night, you will wake up in the morning an *empty vessel.* By the end of each day, your body will demand that you give it a certain amount of fuel (calories), and it will get that fuel, one way or another. When you wake each morning, your body is waiting to be fed and nourished. You can either learn to feed your body *well,* or risk being driven each day to reach for foods that were never designed to help you lose weight. You will also likely eat many of these calories at the worst possible time of the day and well in excess of the calories your body needs.

When you wake up each morning, whatever you may have eaten the day before is gone. Your body has processed the fuel you gave it and spent the duration of your sleeping hours going about its business of repairing muscle cells, replacing damaged cells and generally taking care of you while you are in a state of slumber and are not conscious to take care of yourself.

When you awaken, your body is ready for more fuel. It is ready to be fed. Whether you give your body what it needs is a matter of habit. It is a matter of habit, and it is a matter of conditioning, as well as a matter of decision.

Maybe you're one of the folks who are just too busy to eat when you wake up, and you habitually skip breakfast or maybe grab a cup of coffee on the run. If this is indeed the case, you are already in trouble, maybe not immediately, but trouble's coming somewhere during your day. It may come in the form of too many calories at lunch, or it may come in the form of an overwhelming urge to snack on chips, cookies, or ice cream later in the evening, even after eating too many calories for your evening meal.

Your body will get what it needs one way or another. You can either learn to manage the fuel you consume or your lack of fuel will manage you. There are no two ways about it.

Those who live by The Fitness Response steer their own ship in regard to their fuel intake. They determine the target amount of calories they are going to consume and they **light their metabolic fire**, usually within an hour of rising in the morning.

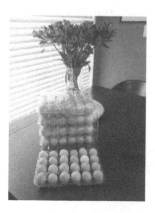

Egg whites are a protein mainstay for bodybuilders and serious fitness enthusiasts

By doing so, the Fitness Responder, puts his or her body to work as soon as the day begins. It is estimated that approximately 10% of the energy *expended* by the body each day is accounted for by the body's processing of food. What does that mean? It means that the work your body does in the process of breaking down the food that you eat is actually a *calorie-burning process.*

Many, many people never capitalize on this fact. People who wake only to skip breakfast and consume their first meal later in the day are making the choice to keep their metabolism in low gear, essentially extending an overnight fast well beyond the 5–8 hours they slept. These people are wasting time!

Serious bodybuilders are masters at keeping their metabolism elevated throughout the day by stoking their metabolic fire with optimal fuel. They understand that the more frequently they eat each day, their body will repay them by burning body fat more consistently and helping them to achieve the lean, muscular shape that we are all accustomed to seeing in these individuals. Doesn't it make sense to model the eating patterns of these people?

Those who eat erratically throughout the day, skipping meals and leaving what they consume to chance, will usually be repaid with excess weight, hunger that is often difficult to tame and a metabolism which has been trained to wait for the excessive calories, which will now be preferentially stored as body fat with ease.

You are an empty vessel. Learn how to fill that vessel in a manner that helps you get the physical results you are after. **Light your metabolic fire** each and every morning. If you don't, you will be at the mercy of a food environment that is not your ally, and you may have a difficult time winning the battle with your weight.

Chapter 6

Carve, Don't Starve (Preempt with Protein)

As I have already mentioned, there is an enormous amount of "food" on the market that is created and produced by man. This food is often low in protein and high in high-glycemic carbohydrate (carbohydrate that tends to rapidly raise blood insulin levels). The fact that we have access to these foods can be viewed as both a blessing and a curse.

In fact, if I were stranded on a desert island and a plane flew overhead accidentally dropping a crate of "snack cakes" and donuts, I would dive in without hesitation. These foods supply a fast, inexpensive means of calories (albeit low nutrient calories) which in some instances serve a positive purpose.

We have all heard stories about some poor individual who accidentally drives their car off into a ravine and finds themselves trapped for days or weeks, only to be rescued alive and well, surviving only by nibbling on some well-known "junk food" found in the car and somehow collecting the nightly accumulation of condensation from the air, preventing their dehydration and ultimate demise.

I am not of the mindset that all "junk food" or "fast food" is bad. People reap the negative results of bad food choices because they make these choices in excess and to the exclusion of healthier choices, more often than not.

I do not support the notion that the restaurant bearing the golden arches is responsible for the obesity crisis we are facing. We are facing this problem because of the chronic repetition with which people make poor food choices, including the choices that come regularly from their local supermarket, and because collectively, we have become more sedentary and less physically active.

Having said this and understanding that much of the manmade and processed foods available to all of us 24/7 are largely sources of high-glycemic' carbohydrate, I will tell you that those who are successful in the fitness and bodybuilding world usually *preempt* their food intake by *targeting a protein* source *first* and foremost.

Please take note: These individuals focus on *feeding their muscle first.*

We know that protein can slow the absorption of glucose or carbohydrate into the bloodstream and that it can quell hunger and prompt the body to rebuild, repair, and optimize muscle.

By eating frequent (every 2–3 hours) meals throughout the day and making sure that the protein content is optimal in each of these meals, relative to the carbohydrate content, you can manage your hunger in a much more effective manner than if you tend to eat high-carbohydrate, low-protein meals.

For those individuals who incorporate resistance exercise (weight lifting or weight training) into a weekly exercise plan, the fact that they are delivering a steady stream of high-quality protein to their system all throughout the day reinforces a trend toward muscle repair, muscle activation, and muscle growth.

Those who follow this dietary rule of thumb (**preempting with protein**), with the desired outcome being weight-loss, can expect that their hunger will likely be much more controlled than if they are in the habit of either skipping breakfast altogether or simply eating two or three high-carbohydrate or low-protein meals throughout the day.

For those individuals whose goal is an increase in muscle mass, muscle tone, muscle definition, or a combination of the three, eating optimal amounts of quality protein at evenly spaced intervals of 2–3 hours throughout the day ensures that they are feeding their muscle at the expense of feeding their body fat.

Because these individuals are usually training and eating in a very specific manner, they can expect that the body will likely respond by increasing its metabolic rate and burning body fat more efficiently, while simultaneously building a desirable amount of lean muscle in the process.

Individuals who are masters at **preempting with protein** usually have a list of protein staples to which they can consistently turn for each and every meal. In the process, they moderate their consumption of higher glycemic carbohydrates.

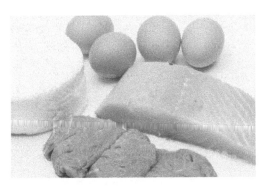

They are well-versed in using high-protein foods such as egg whites, chicken breast, low-fat cottage cheese, turkey breast, soy products, and fish such as tuna, tilapia, and salmon. When they are not in a position to eat their protein with a knife and fork, they often supplement with high-quality sources of protein such as whey and casein found in protein bars or shakes.

If you say, "Ooh, I don't like things like that," you're missing the point. Many people who have achieved the physical best of themselves never woke up in the beginning craving a seven–egg white omelet or a protein shake. These people learned how to use the most nutritious and optimal components of the food that is available to all of us and made the decision to use food as a tool to nourish and change their bodies.

They **preempt with protein** so that they will not be driven to eat the things the rest of us eat without thinking later in the day.

Think about it.

Chapter 7
Add to Your Daily Deficit

For many people, the road to weight-loss is steeped in a long history of deprivation and starvation *alone*. It is true that if weight-loss is to occur in an ongoing and consistent manner, part of what you must strive to do, is to create a calorie deficit, relative to the calories you ingest.

Almost everyone understands on a purely emotional level what the word *diet* means. I think it is fair to say that the mention of the word, for many, surely conjures images of sparsely filled plates of uninteresting food, coupled with a general sense of dread, gloom, and frustration. Many, many dieters tend to approach their weight-loss efforts pitting only their will against the biologically encoded tendency of our bodies to be self-protective against volitional starvation. Given this fact, fighting the weight battle with starvation as the primary tactical approach is a doomed proposition. We all know this. Dieters know this as well.

As I said, your body is designed to protect itself from starvation, from wasting away. Consequently, the body's ability to store calories is an efficient process, particularly where high-glycemic carbohydrate consumption is concerned.

Because our physical bodies were designed to be self-protective, and we in general store excess calories very easily, if you want to lose weight and keep your excess weight off, I encourage you to find ways to **add to your daily deficit**.

For example, if I'm seeing a new patient for the first time and we're discussing the goal-weight that this person wants to achieve, we look at how tall the patient is and determine, based on Body Mass Index and other factors such as waist and hip measurements and body-fat percentage, what an ideal target weight might be. This weight is usually a range, rather than a single number that falls within what would be considered healthy *BMI* (Body Mass Index) based on this persons height.

There are some limitations with the use of BMI as a single measure of an ideal weight; it is not perfect, however, when used with other parameters such as a physical exam by a knowledgeable practitioner, it remains a beneficial tool.

After we determine this target goal weight, I recommend a daily calorie target as well. I encourage the patient not to exceed this target. This calorie intake is usually also a range, as opposed to a strict number. However, the highest calorie intake of that range usually presumes an overall deficit in calories, relative to what patients describe as their usual daily caloric intake. So if I encourage a female patient not to exceed 1400 calories each day, the presumption is that she is likely consuming far more than 1400 calories in her usual, daily diet on a regular basis, particularly if she is gaining weight or struggling to lose excess weight.

Because our goal, when someone needs to lose weight, is to provide a diet that delivers optimal nutrition without starving the patient, we must define a caloric range that delivers adequate calories with optimal nutrition, but which also creates a slight calorie deficit relative to what we estimate the body requires each day for the patient's activities of daily living.

When we have estimated an approximate number of calories that the body needs, we decrease the top-end of the suggested calorie range by 100–200 calories. By doing so, our goal is to deliver optimal nutrition, a reasonable amount of calories each day, but at a slight, relative deficit. We are encouraging the body to meet any additional energy needs by dipping into its store of excess fat.

Now, if my goal were to encourage weight loss by diet alone, that would be the end of it. I might cross my fingers and wish the patient the best of luck. I might pat them on the back as they left my office. However, because I am a strong advocate for lifelong fitness as a component of good health and weight maintenance, my dietary recommendations are almost always made along with a plan for regular, daily exercise.

Daily exercise will invariably differ from person to person; however, even if the recommendation is for a patient to begin a daily walking program, beginning at 5 to 10 minutes per day and working up to 30 to 60 minutes per day, I encourage them to start.

Why is this important? It is important for a several reasons. Number one: **exercise adds to the daily caloric deficit.** Number two: exercise enhances cardiovascular health, improves cognitive function and mental alertness, as well as propagating feelings of wellbeing.

The third reason that exercise is important is that as a daily habit, exercise is one of the primary indicators of people's ability to **maintain their weight loss** after they reach their target or goal weight. It is less likely that someone who loses weight without exercise will suddenly find it important to begin an exercise program, when the foundation for exercise was never laid.

Exercise is like insurance. When life events happen that are outside of our control (a death, a wedding, the holidays, travel, out-of-town guests, etc.), and we are thrown off course, it is much easier to get back on track or lose extra weight gained at the expense of these life occurrences, than might be for someone who does not exercise routinely.

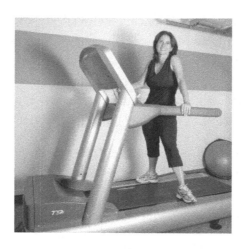

My wife Sherrill, co-owner, fitness consultant, and personal trainer at Physician's Way Healthy Weight Loss in Austin, Texas

If you are just starting out and exercise is not a current part of your life, I encourage you to see your doctor to discuss a reasonable approach to beginning an exercise plan. I have yet to meet another physician who didn't feel that it was in their patients' best interest to lose excess weight.

So no matter what type of dietary or fitness direction you take, see your physician first to ask whether it is a sound approach and to get an opinion as to whether it is a reasonable approach for you.

After your doc gives you the green light to begin, make exercise a daily component of your life and approach to weight-loss. **Add to your daily deficit.** Every step that you take to do so will be additive and it won't be long before your body begins to reflect the positive changes you've been planning as well as hoping to see!

Chapter 8

Total Body Muscle Activation™

After your doctor clears you to begin an exercise program, there are a variety of things to consider. For one, it is important to figure out what you are likely to stick with day after day, week after week, and possibly year after year. It is well-known that most people don't stick to any formal plan of exercise, and those that do are most likely to continue an exercise activity that they enjoy.

So when it comes to making recommendations for daily exercise, we have to keep this fact in mind. It is often said that the best exercise for you is the exercise that you *will* do. In realizing this truth, it can be frustrating for both parties if a physician is trying to convince you to run for 30 minutes to an hour each day, when you simply hate to run. Maybe you would be OK playing tennis three days out of the week, but trying to get you on the track or treadmill will make you both feel like banging your head against a wall.

Regardless, and for the reasons I explained in the preceding chapter, aerobic exercise is beneficial for a variety of reasons. I encourage some form of regular, aerobic activity at least 3 to 4 days per week.

On the other hand, I also want my patients to understand that from a purely calorie burning standpoint, all of the positive aside, while performing aerobic exercise, we are generally **trading time for calories**

burned. Is this a bad thing? If you have the time to spare and you enjoy the activity, it is not. However, aerobic exercise by itself, unless it is sustained for long periods of time, which is not the case for most people, is not the most effective means of creating a physiology that is optimized to more efficiently burn calories while the body is not exercising, or is in a resting state.

I have had countless patients that I see for the first time who tell me, "Doc, I run for an hour and a half, six or seven days a week and I just can't seem to lose any weight at all. I'm stuck!" It might sound hard to believe, but this is not an uncommon complaint. It is also not uncommon for me to meet individuals whose personal trainers or other mentors have demanded that they burn 500 to 1000 calories every day through aerobic exercise, while encouraging them to keep their calorie intake at some arbitrarily low level or putting upon them, unrealistic dietary constraints.

Generally speaking, aerobic exercise may be the only exercise in which these individuals engage. Unfortunately, something that many people don't realize is this: 'Most people *overestimate* how many calories they burn during exercise and *underestimate* the amount of calories they consume.' A pattern in which an individual focuses so much of their time and energy trying to both burn and restrict calories simultaneously, can and often does backfire. Sure, one may lose weight, but at what cost and how long can this pattern be kept up?

For some folks, it may be argued that the fact that they <u>do</u> exercise, may be the reason they gain weight. There may actually be some truth to this statement, in that some of us will actually reward ourselves with food, *because* we engaged in exercise on a particular day, or we'll unknowingly consume more calories than we realize, due to the fact that exercise is known to increase appetite. Certainly I have seen many patients who, despite a steady, rigorous routine of aerobic exercise, simply maintain their weight at a certain point, but don't continue to lose weight.

So how do you create a body and a physiology that burns calories more efficiently and overcomes the limitations of aerobic exercise alone?

The answer is to stimulate and challenge your skeletal muscle through resistance exercise (weight training) on a regular basis.

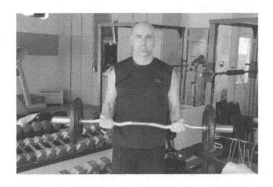

I realize that I may have just lost some of you. Indeed, some people, for whatever reason, are simply averse to the idea of resistance exercise (training with weights). That being said, the benefits of resistance exercise, strength training, weight-lifting or whatever you call it cannot be overstated. Resting muscle is highly metabolically active and burns calories. When challenged through progressive resistance exercise, muscle is activated and stimulated to repair and regenerate. Through this process, two things happen: Muscle becomes stronger, and activated muscle increases the body's metabolic rate, making it possible for the body to burn calories more efficiently, well beyond the period of time that you are engaged in this type of exercise activity.

This reason is in part why men and women in the bodybuilding world, though often more muscular than the average person on the street, can reach very low levels of overall body-fat percentage. These people essentially become calorie-burning machines because of their increased muscle mass, their regular, consistent stimulation of all of their major muscle groups, and the rest and optimal nutrition that allow those muscles to heal and recover.

These individuals are masters at sculpting their physical bodies and decreasing their overall body-fat percentage to very low levels and becoming very lean. Some bodybuilders do very little aerobic exercise, but because of their large amount of activated muscle, they still decrease their overall body fat to such a degree that they remain competitive in their sport (bodybuilding).

If you are interested in optimizing metabolism through resistance exercise and possibly increasing the percentage of muscle you carry, progressive weight-training may be the answer that allows you to break the weight-loss barriers you may have encountered with an aerobics-only exercise program.

In fact, whether people are open to adding this component or not, I at least explain the benefits of resistance exercise to every new patient that I see at my clinic. Some patients are open to this kind of exercise; some are not. For those who are not inclined to add this component, and especially with some women, there may be a fear of "bulking up." This fear is, in general, unfounded. The differences in testosterone level between men and women account for the usual much larger muscle mass found in men.

The fact that some male and female bodybuilders can attain levels of muscle mass well above and beyond that of the average fitness enthusiast is usually more of a testament to highly specific training regimens and more extreme approaches to diet and nutrition (yes, steroid-induced in some cases) than those of the casual, though dedicated fitness enthusiast.

However, it is more apparent than ever that strength or resistance training can benefit people in almost every age range, the very young excluded. In fact, resistance exercise has been shown to keep people stronger, increase bone density, and aid in control of body-fat, well into advanced age.

Because resistance exercise challenges muscle to become stronger and all skeletal muscle attaches to bone to facilitate movement of the body, when muscle is stimulated through training, bone is also stimulated. In this process, bone becomes stronger and denser, which can be a significant factor in preventing the likelihood of a hip or other age related fracture, especially for those who have reached advanced years and may have a family history of osteoporosis.

For the average adult who wants to lose weight and become stronger, leaner, and more fit, I encourage the addition of this component of exercise. By implementing what I call **TBMA**™ or **Total Body Muscle Activation**™ and making a goal of stimulating all major muscle groups on a weekly basis through resistance exercise, you will increase your body's ability to burn calories more efficiently, even outside of the time-related confines of exercise.

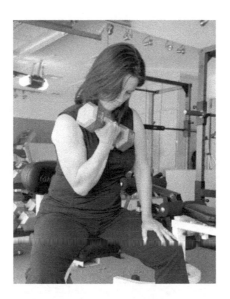

Total Body Muscle Activation™: Utilize it. Embrace it. Let your skeletal muscle bridge the gap where aerobic exercise leaves off. In doing so, you will add a level of control and latitude in your overall ability to burn calories more efficiently, and in the process you will become stronger, leaner, and quite possibly more confident in your ability to take greater control of your physical body, than you may have ever dreamed possible.

Chapter 9

Fuel up!

Day after day I see patients who have no idea why they're struggling to lose weight. They often tell me they've cut back on their calories and only eat once or twice a day.

In fact, why in the world would you not lose weight eating only a couple of times per day? It only seems logical that if you limited your meals to just one or two each day, the weight should fall effortlessly from the body.

However, it just doesn't work that way. The human body is smart. It somehow knows when we are trying to trick or deceive it. If we drastically restrict our calorie intake and decrease the number of meals we eat over the course of the day, the body recognizes this and slows the factory down. Metabolism slows under these circumstances, and the physiologic shift tilts in the direction of fat storage.

If your goal is to lose weight and keep it off, you need to understand that at the most basic level of our beings, we are wired for self-preservation. Our bodies tend to respond to the demands of the environment we are in or the environment that we create. So if you eat irregularly or skip meals, leaving long gaps between the foods you consume, the body will interpret this, in some underlying, mysterious neurological way, as a period of starvation and will slow down your metabolism in an attempt to protect you from wasting away.

You see, your body has no idea how long you will go before you feed again. It just responds to the data and information that you are giving it. If that means that you went to bed at 10 p.m. the previous evening, woke up at 6 a.m., had only a cup of coffee on your way out the door, your first real nutrition being at lunch today, all your body really knows is that it has not been fed for 12–16 hours.

Under these circumstances, your body will go into waiting mode and slow down the physiologic and biochemical pathways that require much energy expenditure. Metabolism slows to protect you from the possibility of breaking down stored body-fat. Again, we are designed for self-preservation. Your body will protect you to an incredible degree when you attempt to starve it.

But something else often occurs when we only eat one or two meals per day. We will often overeat too many calories at the one or two meals we do eat, because we naturally become overly hungry because of the long intervals between meal times. Where weight gain is concerned, this scenario makes the situation even worse because, not only is the body slowing its metabolic rate to protect us from losing body fat or burning calories, now we've taken in an excess of calories in one sitting. The body now actively stores as many calories as possible. If you have been attempting to diet using this infrequent meal strategy, it often backfires just for this reason.

So what do you do to reverse this storage trend? It is just the opposite of what many of us intuitively think. In fact, to encourage the body to liberate stored body fat, we need to eat more frequently, not less frequently.

As I've mentioned before, the digestion of food each day accounts for approximately 10% of the body's overall energy expenditure. Those individuals in the bodybuilding and fitness world intuitively capitalize on this truth. They realize that the food that they eat and the increased frequency and consistency with which they eat, determines how efficient their metabolism will be. They realize that their fat loss is directly tied to how well they eat, not how well they starve themselves. Does this seem a bit counterintuitive? If it does, you are not alone, for many people feel this way.

The point is that we need to accept that this is how the body functions and not ignore reality. If you want to accelerate your metabolic rate, after doing what I encourage in Chapter 5 and "lighting the morning fire," make sure that you consistently feed your body excellent nutrition approximately every 2–3 hours after that first meal of the day. Your body is waiting for you to give it real fuel, and not just that, it is waiting for you to give it really excellent fuel.

As an adult living in the abundant and excessively high-calorie food environment in which we live, eating the traditional large breakfast, lunch, and dinner that so many of us grew up with just doesn't tend to work well for facilitating weight loss. So take a tip from the men and women in the fitness and bodybuilding world who make a science out of feeding themselves the best nutrition they can find; **fuel up** and make sure that you eat great nutrition at intervals of about every 2–3 hours throughout your day. If you do this well, along with a program of daily exercise, your body will repay you by liberating stored body fat. Isn't that what you want?

In the next chapter I will explain how to listen more closely to your body, so that you take in nutrition when your body is calling for it and become more in tune with what your metabolism is trying to tell you.

Chapter 10

Walking the Edge of Hunger™

The number one complaint that I hear from patients when I see them for the first time, is that they are hungry all the time. In fact, because my practice is that of bariatric medicine, I am in a position to use medication to help my patients with appetite control and this is an acceptable modality in my field. Unfortunately, many of these new patients want just one thing and that is for their hunger to *go away*! They feel if they can just not be hungry, they won't eat and their weight will just disappear. I explain to them that *hunger is their metabolism talking to them.*

When we are truly hungry, there is a reason that we feel hungry. Our body is trying to get our attention so that we will take in nourishment. Hunger is a built-in survival mechanism that alerts us to prevent the possibility of starvation. By acknowledging this primal urge and then eating, we assure the body that we are not going to starve it.

We have already acknowledged that the process by which food is broken down and utilized by the body, is a process that burns calories and requires an expenditure of energy to burn these calories. The reason that bodybuilders, athletes, and fitness competitors typically eat 5–6 times during an average day and sometimes even more frequently is that they know this pattern keeps their body's metabolic rate elevated throughout the day and allows the body to burn fat more consistently.

This concept is in sharp opposition to what many dieters believe has to happen for weight-loss to occur.

On the other hand, even though eating small, frequent meals throughout the day tends to allow for greater efficiency where fat burning is concerned, if weight-loss is your ultimate goal, you must consume a reasonable amount of calories each day and not too many.

If we consume more calories than the body needs at any one time, we usually feel it, and the body starts the storage process. We all know what this feels like. Almost everyone knows that feeling when they have eaten more than they intended to, and the couch or recliner is calling.

I encourage my patients to avoid ever eating to the point where they feel this way. Instead, we talk about **walking the edge of hunger**. Approaching one's diet with a plan to walk the edge of hunger is a conscious decision where one eats enough calories during the day to meet ones' basic metabolic needs for good health, but daily calories are spread across at least 5–6 meals, and occasionally more, throughout the day.

When we eat breakfast with the knowledge and understanding that we will be taking in more nutrition again 2–3 hours later, it makes it much easier to eat in moderation, than if we are anticipating only consuming two or three meals during a given day. I explain to my patients that 2–3 hours after eating breakfast or another meal during the day, they should begin to *feel* the slight urge of hunger that should follow if calories weren't overconsumed at the preceding meal.

I want my patients to learn what this feels like and to acknowledge that their metabolism is talking to them and that they should listen closely. By eating just enough calories each meal to get you through the next 2 –3 hours, you learn to walk the edge of hunger and capitalize on the body's natural ability to burn calories more consistently throughout the day. The person that fails to understand that food drives the metabolism is destined to struggle. The last thing that we want to do is snuff out hunger, either with medication or excess food.

Though medication can be useful and beneficial in helping patients navigate the waters of our excessive caloric food environment, I don't use medication to knock out hunger. To do so would defeat the purpose of learning how to manage your metabolism with the use of optimal foods and meal frequency.

Learn to listen to your metabolism. It is talking to you. Learn to listen carefully to what it's telling you and learn to respond in a manner that optimizes your metabolism. If you can learn to do this with consistency, you can develop a physiology that is primed for effective calorie utilization and create a physiologic shift that favors fat loss.

By **walking the edge of hunger**, you will be gaining control over your appetite, while also developing a consciousness about how food affects your body. In the process, you will learn how to utilize food in a way that very few of your peers understand. You will be able to harness the power of what I believe food was always intended to be; fuel.

Chapter 11

Supplement with Protein

In Chapter 6 we talked about preempting with protein as a means of supplying the body's muscle with the building blocks necessary for repair and optimization of that muscle. Please remember that if protein is not sought first, in a given meal, it is often very easy to eat higher levels of starchy carbohydrate than you realize or desire (more about that later).

How much protein is necessary for optimal health has been a point of much controversy between scientists, doctors, and nutrition experts for many years. Fitness and bodybuilding practitioners and enthusiasts generally acknowledge that the U.S. Recommended Daily Allowance (RDA) for protein is simply inadequate. Many physicians and nutritionists echo this line of thought, as well.

The Recommended Daily Allowance for protein consumption is 0.8 grams per kilogram of body weight. This amount, supposedly, is an adequate daily amount of protein for maintenance of general health in an adult. For example, a women whose ideal weight is 130 pounds (or 59 kg) based on RDA recommendations has a daily protein requirement of 59 kg x 0.8 = 47 grams of protein. Is this enough protein to maintain healthy cell growth and repair in an athlete or someone whose goal is the development of greater strength and more muscle; someone who engages in hard physical exercise? It is likely not.

In the fitness world, a women of the same weight who wants to increase her muscle mass and improve her overall strength might consume a daily amount of protein closer to 1.5 to 2 grams of protein per pound of her target or goal weight. So, if she ultimately wanted to gain 5 pounds of muscle, with a resulting weight of 135 pounds, she might take in anywhere between 202 to 270 grams of protein per day, or possibly even more.

She would eat this amount to complement her resistance training program and to increase the delivery of a steady stream of amino acids (the breakdown product of protein) to the muscles to assure muscle repair and growth.

How much protein is too much? This question is controversial, to say the least. Some physicians fear that excess protein could overload or damage the kidneys or other organs. In fact, people with kidney, liver, or other health issues should always consult their physician to determine how much protein is reasonable in their particular situation.

On the other hand, there is likely a wide range of protein that can be consumed safely by an individual in good health. In fact, if we look at cultures such as the Eskimos, their diet has historically relied mostly on meat and fats derived from fish, seals, whales, and other creatures from the land and sea.

An Internet article from the archives of *TIME* magazine, dated Monday, May 18, 1936 reported this: Eskimos do not suffer from diabetes or cancer, rarely from hardening of the arteries. Yet they subsist almost entirely on meat. The article went on to say:

> …When food is abundant, a healthy Eskimo living under primitive conditions will eat 5 to 10 pounds of meat a day." Trappers rely on caribou and dried buffalo meat. Hunters eat seal, walrus and whale meat. The Eskimo "has some carbohydrates for approximately two months in the year, in the

form of blueberries. He also relishes the stomach contents of the caribou which, throughout the year, contain carbohydrates… The stomach contents are often eaten with seal oil—a salad! When an Eskimo catches a walrus, he immediately opens the stomach and eats all of the clams… The Eskimos eat the livers of practically all animals, except that of the white bear… Only when in need does he consume very large quantities of fat. Blubber is not regarded as a delicacy." That diet supplies all the proteins, fats and carbohydrates which the Eskimos need to thrive on. Whenever they adopt white men's flour, they develop alkalosis.

In fact, as the Eskimos have adopted many of the highly processed convenience foods and products from the influx of Western civilization, dental and physical ailments that were practically nonexistent in the early part of the 20th century, have become widespread and common, arguably secondary to their increased consumption of processed sources of carbohydrate.

So how much protein is too much? There is no pat answer to this question, but suffice to say, we likely consume far less than we could, especially for the development of optimal health and fitness.

Because I truly believe the body functions at its best when we graze on smaller, highly nutritious meals throughout the day and because a steady stream of amino acids in the bloodstream allows for optimization of muscle, finding supplemental sources of protein can make meeting one's protein needs much simpler, as well as more convenient.

For an individual who does routinely engage in rigorous exercise and includes strength or resistance training in their program, there are many excellent sources of supplemental protein on the market from which to choose.

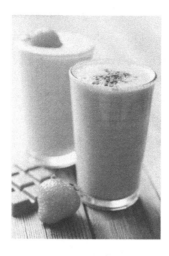

Meal replacement with supplemental protein can take at least some of the guess work out of planning one's day, from the standpoint of attempting to eat for optimal nutrition. Choosing many of these protein sources may allow you to target a specific range of daily protein, without every meal being derived from animal flesh. This consideration is more important to some people than others, but the point is that using supplemental protein can provide you with more dietary options and convenience, as well.

Whether you choose to supplement with protein or not, understand that doing so is certainly a common practice for many athletes, fitness enthusiasts, and often a given for those who practice bodybuilding.

Note that there are *complete* as well as *incomplete* sources of protein. A complete protein source, such as animal protein (meat, fish, chicken, eggs), contains all of the amino acids that the body requires for muscle growth and general cell repair. Incomplete protein sources, such as vegetables, nuts, seeds, and grains, provide some, but not all, of the amino acids required for cell building and repair. A diet that provides a variety of plant and animal products will most likely supply all the necessary amino acids the body needs for good health, but not necessarily optimal amounts of quality protein to meet the needs of someone who trains their body in a serious, goal-oriented manner.

There are many different sources of supplemental protein on the market, and I am not going to advocate any one brand or form over another. However, here are just some of the types of protein you might consider if you choose to expand beyond whole foods to meet your protein needs:

- **Whey Protein**: Whey is derived from milk and has been long considered the standard when it comes to protein supplementation. Whey protein is a fast-releasing protein which rapidly provides the bloodstream a pool of amino acids and makes for an excellent pre or post workout meal replacement which can aid in more rapid repair and recovery of the muscle cells. Whey can be found in packaged protein bars and shakes and also in powder form.

- **Soy Protein**: Soy is a plant-based protein (from soy beans) that supplies a complete source of amino acids. Studies show it to be an effective source for repair and preservation of lean muscle.

- **Casein Protein**: Casein is also derived from milk. Because it is slower to digest than whey protein, it is an excellent protein source to consider before bedtime, because it tends to break down slowly during the night, providing a steady stream of amino acids for the body to use in repairing and optimizing muscle during sleep.

- **Egg Protein**: This protein is derived from the white or albumin portion of eggs. Egg protein is an excellent source of essential amino acids and is easily absorbed and used by the body for muscle building and repair. Many forms are on the market, from whole egg sources, to packaged egg whites to powdered forms of egg protein.

There are other protein products. These are but a handful of the types of supplemental protein sources from which to choose and you may find that there are many different brands of each type on the market. If your goal is to consume optimal fuel throughout each day in an effort to more fully support physical change through exercise and training, adding supplemental protein sources can enhance and simplify meeting your daily protein needs.

When you routinely eat at least 5–6 small, nutritious meals each day to keep metabolism elevated, planned protein supplementation can ease the challenge all serious fitness enthusiasts face, in choosing to eat in a more frequent manner.

I have no doubt that protein supplementation can be beneficial in the pursuit of helping to facilitate positive physical change within the context of a dedicated, goal oriented training program. Protein supplementation is akin to putting jet fuel into a jet. In truth, we all need to eat. Those seeking the physical changes that come only with specific, targeted physical training will require a highly nutritious, optimal daily diet.

Choosing to consume a quality protein bar or shake at any point in your day is a conscious decision to *not* eat something less nutritious in that moment. Only jet fuel will efficiently run the engine of a jet. Consequently, high-quality protein is the best way to feed your muscle and give your body the amino acids it requires to optimize and repair that muscle.

We have all had the urge when hunger calls to head to a vending machine or through a fast food drive-through. I encourage you to be smart about your diet with each and every choice that you make. **Supplement with good, quality protein**, especially when you're tempted to make a poor dietary choice instead. As you watch your body's response to your efforts over time, you will know that you are headed in the right direction and that you are giving your body the best possible fuel that you can, day after day.

Chapter 12

Stay Off of the Carbo-coaster

The consumption of food exerts powerful influence over our bodies. So the more you understand about food, the more control you have over the impact of food on your body.

If you are a women who has ever been pregnant and under the care of a physician, you may be familiar with a test which is done routinely, called the *glucose tolerance test*. The *glucose tolerance test* is usually performed somewhere between the second and third trimester of pregnancy. This test is also frequently used to diagnosis diabetes, insulin resistance, or reactive hypoglycemia.

The *glucose tolerance test* is performed by giving a fasting patient an oral glucose solution to drink, then drawing blood glucose levels, depending on the type of testing being done, at time zero, 1 hour, 2 hours and 3 hours to determine how the body processes and clears the bloodstream of excess glucose.

Because physiology in pregnancy is altered in various ways, one concern is that the pregnant patient can develop gestational diabetes (diabetes of pregnancy), whereby circulating blood glucose remains higher than normal. This state can cause a variety of pathologic states in both the mother and the baby, if not dealt with during the pregnancy.

Glucose tolerance testing shines a light on the how efficiently the body clears excessive glucose from the bloodstream over a relatively short period of time.

In persons (males included) who are not pregnant and who are not diabetic, the process by which the body clears excess glucose is an extremely efficient one. The fact that this process is so efficient is the main reason that you need more of an understanding of the macronutrients from which food is made, how certain foods affect your body, and why it is difficult to view food solely as "points," as do certain purely dietary approaches.

Food is composed of three macronutrients that fuel the body in different ways. Those macronutrients are *fats, carbohydrates,* and *proteins.* Food can be composed solely of any of these by themselves. For example, a stick of butter is essentially pure fat, as is a bottle of olive oil. Food can also be composed of a combination of macronutrients:

- A rib-eye steak is an example of a food product that is mostly protein, but also has visible fat mixed in with negligible, but present carbohydrate.

- Pasta is an example of a food that is largely carbohydrate, but may contain small amounts of fat and protein.

- An avocado is mostly composed of fat, but also has a percentage of both protein and carbohydrate.

Food is often a combination of these three macronutrients, frequently with one macronutrient being the most prominent.

Knowing this, allows individuals who are trying to lose weight or transform their physical appearance through optimal nutrition and exercise, the ability to make more strategic food choices, which they know, often through trial and error, will yield the positive changes that they are seeking.

Understanding the components of the foods that you choose to eat on a day-to-day basis becomes especially important with manmade or highly processed foods, because the most inexpensive macronutrients used in the food industry are usually fats and carbohydrates.

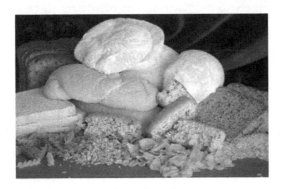

The combinations in which fat and carbohydrate can be paired from the standpoint of food production, is mind-boggling. Many of the processed foods that are available today also contain much less protein per unit or serving than the amount of fat and carbohydrate which they possess. This ratio becomes even more significant in light of the fact that over the past 30 years or so, the food industry has responded to the tide of public sentiment, generated by fuzzy research data and a governmental push to make fat enemy number one in the war against both obesity and heart disease.

Because fat has become the vilified, evil macronutrient to avoid, food manufacturers have responded over the past 30 years by drastically lowering the overall fat content of the foods they produce. We have all seen the labels for "low-fat or low cholesterol" on box labels of all kinds of products.

This shift in food production that decreases fat content in already low-protein containing food products, results in an overall increase in the high-glycemic carbohydrate content of these foods. It has become painfully clear that this shift has not made a dent in our overweight and obesity problem. Why? It comes back to what I explained previously:

The body's ability to breakdown and process carbohydrates is extremely efficient. When the body processes carbohydrate, whether from simple sugars such as found in a soda or from a bowl of pasta, its ultimate destination is largely to fat storage, unless the body is engaged in an activity that is likely to use these sugars before fat storage occurs.

Gary Taubes, science writer and author of *Good Calories, Bad Calories*, explains it like this, in his latest book, *Why We Get Fat, And What to Do about It*:

> As it turns out, two factors will essentially determine how much fat we accumulate, both having to do with the hormone insulin. First, when insulin levels are elevated, we accumulate fat in our fat tissue; when these levels fall, we liberate fat from the fat tissue and burn it for fuel. This has been known since the early 1960s and has never been controversial. Second, our insulin levels are effectively determined by the carbohydrates we eat—not entirely, but for all intents and purposes. The more carbohydrates we eat, the easier they are to digest and the sweeter they are, the more insulin we will secrete, meaning that the level of it in our bloodstream is greater and so is the fat we retain in our fat cells. "Carbohydrate is driving insulin is driving fat," is how George Cahill, a former professor of medicine at Harvard Medical School, recently described this to me. Cahill had done some of the early research on the regulation of fat accumulation in the 1950s, and then he coedited an eight-hundred-page American Physiological Society compendium of this research that was published in 1965.

> In other words, the science itself makes clear that hormones, enzymes, and growth factors regulate our fat tissue, just as they do everything else in the human body, and that we do not get fat because we overeat, we get fat because the carbohydrates in our diet make us fat. The science tells us that obesity is ultimately the result of a hormonal imbalance, not

a caloric one—specifically, the stimulation of insulin secretion caused by eating easily digestible, carbohydrate-rich foods: refined carbohydrates including flour and cereal grains, starchy vegetables such as potatoes, and sugars, like sucrose (table sugar) and high fructose corn syrup. These carbohydrates literally make us fat, and by driving us to accumulate fat, they make us hungrier and the make us sedentary.

This is the fundamental reality of why we fatten, and if we're to get lean and stay lean, we'll have to understand and accept it, and, perhaps more important, our doctors are going to have to understand and acknowledge it, too.

Those in the fitness world, particularly bodybuilders, know that the ingestion of protein, along with carbohydrate tends to slow the absorption of carbohydrate, potentially limiting what might otherwise be a more rapid rise in insulin level. Protein consumption is also well known to offer longer periods of satiety, than does carbohydrate.

Bodybuilders and those who have a strong understanding of how the macronutrients of food affect the body capitalize on the fact that protein increases satiety. They tend toward a dietary approach that usually contains higher-than-average levels of protein, paired with more moderate or lower amounts of high-glycemic carbohydrate. These calories are usually spread across five or more meals throughout the day. By doing so, these individuals can strategically temper the fat-storing tendency that tends to naturally follow eating high-carbohydrate, low-protein meals.

Aside from offering increased satiety, dietary protein is the only macronutrient that has been shown to enhance the possibility of weight-loss when this component of food is increased in the diet. It is well known to physiologists that protein has a higher TEF (Thermic Effect of Food), meaning that the body uses a higher percentage of calories to process protein than it uses to process either dietary fat or carbohydrate.

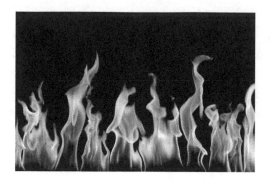

Your Metabolism is fueled by food!

Serious athletes and bodybuilders understand that at the most basic level, muscle is made of protein. The ingestion of dietary protein has been shown to promote *protein turnover*. For those who engage in regular resistance training, this translates into muscle repair, which then translates into muscle growth and elevated metabolic rate secondary to the increased activity of activated lean muscle.

By focusing on eating lean sources of protein with moderate levels of dietary carbohydrate and fat, fitness athletes and bodybuilders take control to a greater degree, of the way they allow food to affect their bodies. Does this practice seem obsessive? Some may argue that is indeed the case. On the other hand, so many people spend years and years in frustration and heartache, obsessing on food and feeling hungry and deprived because they have no idea how to manage food effectively.

I see these patients day after day in my practice. Many of them report that they are starving all day long and that all they can think about is food. Does that sound obsessive? As I glance at their written dietary journals, what is completely allusive to them becomes very obvious to me.

High-glycemic carbohydrate is like a drug. Consumption of unopposed carbohydrate (carbohydrate ingested without protein) tends to be digested very quickly, leading to an overreaching insulin response and a rapid storage of blood glucose. This is followed by the return of what can often be excessive hunger, even an hour or so later.

So when my patients tell me that they are "starving," I ask them what they had for breakfast that day. I am never surprised when they tell me, "I had a bagel and a banana" or "I had a bowl of cereal" or I had a "granola bar."

Eating unopposed carbohydrate will earn you a surefire ticket on the *carbo-coaster*, whereby you have created a physiologic cycle which is driving you to seek out the next fast sugar-fix only hours away from your last meal.

I explain to my own patients that those in the fitness world, who are good at getting to where they want to go, physically speaking, rarely eat in a manner that leads to a ride on the **carbo-coaster.**

What's the take-home message here? If you want to get good at losing weight and to take control of your body, you must take the time to learn what the foods you eat are made of and then learn to eat them in a more strategic manner.

In the most basic sense, food is fuel and that's all. This does not mean that eating logically can't taste good or be extremely enjoyable. What we as humans spend our day eating is a matter of learned behavior and habit.

In our clinic, we talk about eating *lean and green*. In the fitness world, this is called eating *clean*. Either way, it's about learning how to fuel your body in the most optimal manner to yield the results you truly want.

Commit to managing both your simple and starchy carbohydrate consumption. In the process, you will learn to manage your most powerful fat-storage hormone, <u>insulin</u>, a hormone which you have the ability, by food choices you make, to influence to a great degree, day-in and day-out.

Stay off the carbo-coaster. Think about the foods you routinely put in your mouth. Learn to eat these foods in a logical and strategic manner. The more you understand what your food is made of, the greater control you will exert in the process of making lasting changes.

Chapter 13
Lose the Booze

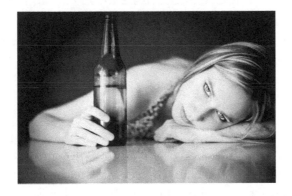

Ok, let's face it: many of us are partial to a little nip now and again. We live in a world that relaxes, celebrates, and grieves with alcohol. For some folks, alcohol is a rare and occasional indulgence and for others a daily occurrence.

In medical school, I was taught that when asking people how much alcohol they typically drink, to take that figure and multiply by three. The prevailing assertion is that most people when asked, are prone to "misrepresent" how frequently and how much they imbibe.

I can't tell you how many completely drunk individuals I have cared for in the emergency department over the years who told me; "I've only had two beers tonight," which usually prompts the response from the surrounding medical team, "They must have been two really big beers!"

For a variety of reasons, we don't always tell the truth about how much we drink.

I can tell you, however, that regular or irregular excessive use of alcohol can and very often does slow the process of one's efforts to lose weight.

It's true that the moderate, thoughtful use of alcohol has been shown by certain research studies to have some positive health benefits, specifically, benefiting cardiovascular health and possibly decreasing the risk of heart attack and stroke, as alcohol may contribute to inhibition of blood clot formation, due to its effect on the blood platelets. On the other hand, excessive alcohol use has a variety of potential health risks, weight gain being just one.

I explain to my patients that alcohol in excess decreases their motivation to exercise, slows metabolism, increases the possibility of accidental injury to self or others, leads to weight gain through empty calories in the alcohol itself, as well as leading to dietary inhibition, whereby one makes poor food choices when alcohol is on board.

If you are serious about losing weight and changing your body, you must temper your use of alcohol. The American Heart Association makes this recommendation:

> If you drink alcohol, do so in moderation. This means an average of one to two drinks per day for men and one drink per day for women. (A drink is one 12 oz. beer, 4 oz. of wine, 1.5 oz. of 80-proof spirits, or 1 oz. of 100-proof spirits.) **Drinking more alcohol increases such dangers as alcoholism, high blood pressure, obesity, stroke, breast cancer, suicide and accidents. Also, it's not possible to predict in which people alcoholism will become a problem. Given these and other risks, the American Heart Association cautions people NOT to start drinking ... if they do not already drink alcohol.**

Consult your doctor on the benefits and risks of consuming alcohol in moderation.

From a strictly weight-loss perspective, the less you consume alcohol the better. Individuals who are serious about changing the composition of their bodies through exercise and optimal nutrition often have little use for alcohol in their life.

If you are consuming alcohol in excess on a regular basis, do yourself a favor and **lose the booze.** You may find that eliminating this singular source of calories helps you to turn the corner in your effort to lose weight and increases your overall level of health and fitness, self-confidence, and self-esteem. In doing so, you may also find that you have more clarity regarding the pursuit of your health and fitness goals. You may achieve your goals much quicker than if alcohol remains a priority in your life.

If you feel that the elimination of this habit is something you can't seem to do alone or maybe you already know that you need help with this issue, there are many organizations out there which provide counseling services and treatment. I encourage you to contact your own physician, if necessary, as they can guide you in a direction that can provide help, if you need it.

Chapter 14

Don't Reward Yourself

Those of us fortunate enough to live in the United States we literally live within the midst of a cornucopia. At almost any hour of the day or night, most of us have access to any number of fast food restaurants, diners, pizza delivery companies and a myriad of supermarkets and convenience stores. There are pubs, bar and grills, and restaurants specializing in everything from beer and Buffalo wings to all-you-can-eat Mexican, Italian, Chinese, and Indian food in cities all throughout our great land.

Access to this kind of culinary variety is wonderful on many levels. However, it also predisposes us to a mentality that informs us that life can be a party pretty much anytime that we want it to be.

Many of us leave work with coworkers at lunchtime and gather at the local all-you-can-eat Chinese buffet. We are offered decadent deserts after lunch and possibly alcohol with any meal of the day. We literally have it all, and in so many ways, we are truly blessed.

On the other hand, if your goal is to change and improve your body, sculpt your physique, and achieve lean muscle definition, this result comes only through consistent nutrition and hard work. You must distance yourself from the party or at least the party that seems to spring from the day-to-day necessity of dining out with your coworkers.

By the same token, if you are serious about achieving the best of yourself, physically, then you literally must guard against the party mentally at any moment in the day. This may mean avoiding the donuts that your boss or office mate brings in almost daily or the afternoon ice cream social which may be promoted by management to bring its employees together.

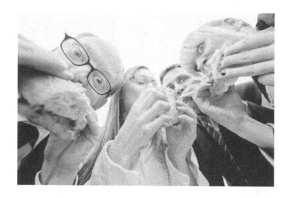

Avoiding unplanned, highly concentrated calories at random times in the day is usually high on the list of those individuals who incorporate The Fitness Response into their lives.

Those among us who are struggling to lose weight may have the mindset that I've alluded to previously, that they exercise a few days each week, but with the full intention of rewarding their efforts with food. This reward may not even be a conscious, planned act. Rather, when an opportunity presents itself (a coworker brings in a chocolate cake), people may succumb to the temptation, if they are not fully focused on the correlation between their dietary and nutrition plan, as it relates to their daily exercise. They may dive into the cake, because mentally, they have negotiated the fair exchange between the effort they have already exerted through exercise and their now, deserved reward.

The greatest problem with this scenario is that it tends to be a repetitive trend for many people. We already know that we often overestimate the calories we burn through exercise, and we tend to underestimate the number of calories we consume. As an ongoing trend, the tendency to reward oneself for exercise is a bad one. In my own practice, I have a pretty good sense of the patients who fall into this exercise-reward pattern. Their results are never consistent, and their weight tends to fluctuate quite a bit. One month they may be down 5 pounds, and the following month they're back up 7 pounds. These patients are generally frustrated with their lack of consistent results, and I very often am too.

We have all heard the phrase, "Nothing tastes as good as thin feels" or "Nothing tastes as good as fit feels." But we all know that in the moment, food can be extremely enticing and powerful. What those foods happen to be differ from person to person, but we all have our temptations. I love Buffalo wings, and they always seem better with a cold beer to accompany them. For so many others, it may be candy, cookies, cakes, and desserts that they have difficulty staying away from.

Motivational guru Anthony Robbins talks about the pain-pleasure principle; that we tend to do things in any moment with the unconscious goal of gaining pleasure or avoiding pain. For those who smoke, many will say that they do so because "It calms me down or decreases my stress." For some people, a few hours in the office leads to pent-up tension, boredom, or anxiety, and they may seek relief from the *pain* of the moment, by stepping outside for a smoke.

Some of us use food to relieve tension, stress, or boredom or to gain pleasure in a certain moment, but in doing so, just like the smoker, we are affecting our health and usually not for the positive.

The idea of implementing The Fitness Response is to gain control over what you put in your mouth because a higher goal is at stake. Yes, some will argue that being so regimented with food and focusing so much on ones' body is obsessive. Maybe it is to some degree, but so is the extreme opposite of being obsessed with high calorie, poor nutrient, high-fat food. The implications of leading a fitness-focused life versus the implications of living a food-focused life can be dramatic. The national overweight and obesity statistics bear this out. We are collectively in trouble and need to do something to change the course we're on.

You are the only one that can change you. On the other hand, we do have the power to influence each other with our actions. I want to encourage you to use The Fitness Response in your own life and **don't reward yourself** for the fact that you exercised today, yesterday, or last week.

Your reward will come incrementally as you consistently use food for what it was intended to be, fuel. Your reward will ultimately be better health along with a body that you are happy with and a body that feels great to be your own.

As an advocate and practitioner of The Fitness Response, I can attest to the fact that "Nothing tastes as good as fit feels." Though I sometimes give in to temptation, it never feels all that great, after the fact.

Do yourself a favor: **Don't reward yourself** with food. It's counterproductive to your goals, and the trade-off just isn't worth it.

Chapter 15

Eat Strategically

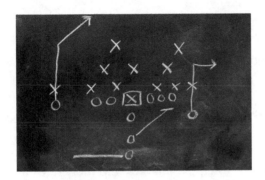

Eight dangerous words are uttered by millions upon millions of people every single day and because of these words, millions and millions of pounds will be gained throughout the land. We probably we have all uttered these words, but how frequently that you do so can have devastating consequences to your weight.

The words I'm talking about are, "Where do you want to go for lunch?" Sure, this phrase may seem innocent enough, but in a country where you can have a smorgasbord at any and all hours of the day or night, this phrase can leave you wide open for trouble.

If you are seriously committed to losing weight and reaching an optimal level of fitness, you must beware of the uncertainty of purpose that these words can open up for you. If you want to reach a physical goal that few seem able to achieve, you must refuse to eat like the masses.

Those in the fitness community, whose mindset is honed like a laser on reaching the best of themselves, physically, tend to not leave lunch or any other meal to chance or to the whims of their coworkers.

If you don't want to look like the pack, you must decline to dine like the pack, unless your goal is to pack on the pounds. In fact, the idea that scores upon scores of people journey out from the office at noon together, their destination an all-you-can-eat buffet or its equivalent, is a sad commentary on where we've arrived today. For many in our society, we don't dine out so much for nutrition anymore, as much as we do for volume and for convenience.

I am going to presume that you are on a different path. So consequently, I am going to recommend that you model your approach to daily diet along the lines of those individuals who have achieved an outcome similar to one that you want.

In my clinic, Physician's Way Healthy Weight Loss in Austin, TX, I encourage my patients to eat "lean and green." In the fitness world, this is equivalent to eating "clean" and is about focusing on good quality sources of protein, vegetables, and moderate amounts of starchy carbohydrate. For those focused on achieving and maintaining their fittest, healthiest body, eating clean is a way of life, and there is usually much rhyme and reason to when and what these people eat throughout any given day.

Individual approach may vary and usually does from person to person; however, there may be some common threads that are shared among many who choose to **eat strategically**. For instance, one common strategic eating maneuver among fitness enthusiasts might be to do aerobic exercise in the morning on an empty stomach, allowing 30 to 60 minutes to pass before eating breakfast, and possibly going lower at this meal on starchy forms of carbohydrate than on a resistance training day.

The bias or belief here is that you are manipulating the body to dip into fat storage to meet any energy needs required during your morning aerobic exercise, because this exercise is being done in a fasting state (you have been asleep all night and awaken with an empty stomach). Thirty to sixty minutes are allowed to pass without eating following exercise, with the intent of allowing the body to equilibrate to its pre-exercise state while forcing the body to meet energy needs by dipping into fat storage.

Some individuals using this maneuver might also keep their carbohydrate level lower on the next one or two of their following meals with the intent of encouraging the body towards a prolonged period of fat catabolism. A note of caution: you really need to be in tune with your body in doing this, because it is easy, due to inexperience with this type of strategic eating pattern, to undershoot your need for carbohydrate and find yourself light-headed or faint. I personally don't recommend that you eat very low or no carbohydrate beyond the first meal of the day. There are exceptions to this stance, but we'll talk about them shortly.

Another approach to **strategic eating** might be to simply make sure that on days you are performing resistance exercise or strength training, that you do have a source of carbohydrate (possibly a starchy form of carbohydrate) at each of your five or six meals of the day. You will then ensure that your muscles have adequate stored glycogen to meet the energy needs required for the demands of strength training. (Glycogen is a store of carbohydrate in the liver and muscle, released as glucose when needed by the body.) Some individuals actually schedule their resistance or strength training for later in the day, as opposed to the morning, to ensure that their muscles are adequately loaded with glycogen, in an attempt to optimize their training on a given day.

When weight-loss is a main priority while in the pursuit of fitness, I often encourage my patients to back off of starchy forms of carbohydrate over the last two meals of the day and encourage more fibrous forms of carbohydrate (vegetables) instead. For the sixth or final meal of the day, I generally encourage more of a pure protein meal, such as chicken breast, egg-whites or cottage cheese, lean beef or a meal replacement protein bar or shake.

This approach to the last two meals of the day ensures that you are not giving your body sources of carbohydrate in the form of starches or simple sugars, which the body easily converts to stored body fat. Eating a pure protein meal before bedtime, for those who engage in regular, weekly strength training, is a **strategic eating maneuver** designed to give the body a steady stream of amino acids during the night's sleep, which the body can use for optimization and repair of muscle tissue.

The last piece of advice I will give along these lines is a general one. We have all heard the sage advice to "eat breakfast like a king, eat lunch like a prince, and dinner like a pauper." Though I don't advocate overeating at any meal, and I advise spreading your calories out over multiple small meals each day, I do believe that one of the wisest **strategic eating moves** that you can make, especially when it comes to managing your weight, is to wind down your calories as the day is ending.

In fact, the further you are away from the time you exercised, and the closer you are to bedtime, the fewer calories it makes sense to ingest. Be very mindful of what you allow to cross your lips after 6 p.m. I am not saying, "Don't eat." Rather, be careful of high-calorie food and drink. This tends to be the bewitching time of the day, when many of us are prone to dietary transgressions we will regret the following day.

Also, as mentioned before, watch your alcohol intake. Many people come home from work, school, or other daily obligations and use alcohol to relax. We have already talked about this topic, but again, drinking alcohol is an easy way to take in unnecessary empty calories that often lead us to further dietary indiscretion. Be mindful if you drink alcohol.

Keep these things in mind as you approach tomorrow. Plan to eat strategically. Don't allow the whims of your friends, coworkers, or anyone else to throw you off course. Our bodies are a reflection of what we do consistently, from the standpoint of both nutrition and exercise.

Whatever you do, stay away from the all-you-can-eat buffets. This one strategy can save you thousands of calories in one sitting. Learn to **eat strategically** and stay the course. In doing so, you will literally separate yourself from the crowd, and you will be happy and proud of the new you that you are becoming.

Chapter 16
Cheat Occasionally

"But, Dr. Kelley, I can't eat like this every single day, I'd go crazy." "I mean, I just can't live without a slice of caramel truffle cheesecake delight every now and then!"

We've all got our own unique cravings for food or drink that we just seem to gravitate to from time to time and that we are unlikely to bypass in the moment. For some it may be sugary sweet desserts, for others savory, hearty, or salty and crunchy, but there is usually some food that calls to us all.

Take heart and note that even the pros grab a *cheat meal* or dessert here and there as a strategic dietary tactic that actually helps to keep them on track. Amateur and professional bodybuilders alike often plan to take either a cheat meal or for some, a cheat day, to keep them on track and to ensure that they have the mental fortitude to stay the course for the long run.

"But, Dr. Kelley, didn't you say not to reward myself?" Yes, I did. However, there is a marked difference here. In one instance, we are talking about someone who is exercising and following a stringent nutrition plan, day after day, only to interrupt that pattern for a well-thought-out cheat to help them stay the course. In Chapter 14, I was referring to the pattern that many fall into, whereby nutrition and exercise are inconsistent to begin with and where the very act of exercise is used to earn someone the validation to reward themselves in a random, less-than-thoughtful manner.

To a dieter, having a cheat meal may be an act that resurrects feelings of guilt and personal wrongdoing, but for those individuals who know and understand that they are using a particular cheat meal or cheat day as an intentional and strategic maneuver, designed to quell urges for something beyond egg whites and grilled chicken breast, it elicits no such guilt and in fact, can be very pleasurable, reassuring, and rewarding.

Some bodybuilders cheat on a weekly basis, taking one meal each week and eating just about anything that they want or that they've been denying themselves in the course of towing the line consistently 6 days in a row before cheating. This meal may be pizza, enchiladas, Buffalo wings and beer, cheesecake, or a big steak and a baked potato, but it is something that is not on the usual daily menu of the serious fitness devotee. Others cheat less frequently, but those who accept and incorporate the cheat meal or cheat day as a tool, generally benefit by gaining more control to stay the course that they have chosen, in pursuit of a better body.

There is also a commonly held notion that in cheating, an individual who is training hard day-in and day-out, may actually be supplying the body with nutrients from the cheat day or cheat meal that possibly may have been excluded to some extent by following their usual strict, clean diet.

It is also not uncommon for those who train their bodies in a rigorous and consistent manner to find that they actually lose a few pounds or that their body fat percentage drops a bit the day following a cheat. Some believe this is possible because the cheat day or cheat meal somehow reinforces to the body that there is no danger of starvation or deprivation of nutrients. Regardless of what the body actually "thinks," it often responds, for the bodybuilder or serious fitness athlete, in a positive manner. Thus the act of cheating on a regular basis is reinforced by visible or measurable physical change.

One of the greatest benefits of cheating, however, is strictly mental. As I noted previously, we all have foods that we know we can't eat on a daily basis and expect that we will continue to lose weight, if that is our goal. However, knowing that the opportunity is there for you to indulge in some culinary delight at regular, well-spaced intervals is comforting to know and anticipate.

Cheating gives reinsurance to our brain that all of our hard work is followed at some point by a positive payoff. For many individuals, bodybuilding is not a hobby; it is an ongoing lifestyle and one that requires a long-term vision and unending dedication to the craft. These are individuals who at some point made the decision that having an average physique was just not OK with them.

These individuals don't take lightly the fuel they put into their bodies. Ninety-nine percent of the time, they may eat in a highly focused, unerring manner. However, they also understand how to use to their benefit, foods that others may view as a dietary indiscretion, in an ongoing effort to stay the course.

If you are on the path of seeking physical transformation or simply an ongoing improvement in your physique, focus on eating clean most of the time. Your efforts will not go unrewarded. On the other-hand, **cheat occasionally** and let your brain and body know that there is a payoff for your efforts. Done strategically, rather than feeling guilty afterwards, you may find that you have a renewed sense of satisfaction, as opposed to deprivation. You may also find that you have a stronger resolve to pursue the road you've chosen to travel.

Chapter 17

Act Like a Pro

In reading the chapter on The Fitness Response™, it may be obvious to you that I believe there are basic, notable differences in the lifestyles between those individuals who tend to progress, lose weight and get fit, versus those of individuals who fail to progress or make limited progress toward improving their bodies.

If I can encourage you to make one major shift in your approach to your weight, your health and your overall fitness, it is this: Stop thinking and looking at this process as something you do occasionally. Your state of health and fitness should not be a periodic endeavor.

I see patients everyday who tell me how they have struggled with their weight all of their lives. This is truly painful and heart wrenching to hear. However, they also tell me, "I just want to lose 25 pounds because I have a reunion coming up" or "I lose 15 pounds by dieting and exercise, but I always put it back on." When I ask, "Why do you think you put the weight back on?" The answer is almost always the same: "Well, I stopped exercising and started eating the way I did before the diet."

We tend to address our health only when there are problems. Excess weight tends to be no different.

I want to encourage you to get out of the mindset that fitness, even optimal fitness, is not important. If you are overweight, the likelihood that taking your dog for a walk three nights each week is going to result in significant weight loss is pretty slim in my experience.

I am going to challenge you to **act like a pro** where your daily diet and exercise are concerned. Resolve that you are going to begin a *daily* exercise program, and that your diet is going to be in *response* to the fact that you did and do exercise daily.

This idea may seem a completely foreign concept to some, however, you must realize that our physical bodies are a reflection of what we do consistently. Our bodies reflect our consistent lack of exercise, as well as the quality of the food and the specificity of the food we consistently deliver to ourselves.

Begin to **act like a pro**, and hold yourself accountable to getting in shape and staying there. Part of acting like a pro means that you can't let other activities or responsibilities get in the way of doing what you know you need to do each and every day.

The fact that people often give 10, 12, and sometimes 14 hours to a job each day and not give themselves at least 30 minutes each day to stimulate their metabolism through exercise is insane in my opinion, if not on some level, irresponsible. Patients who are dangerously obese tell me all the time, "I just don't have time to exercise." I will often tell them, "You don't have the luxury of <u>not</u> taking the time to exercise."

Our priorities are so distorted when it comes to placing value on our health and on maintaining it. We frequently give away our time to others, often in exchange for little of value, and we cheat ourselves, robbing ourselves of something that is truly invaluable: our optimal health.

Think about it: Walking is free. We could get out and walk almost daily, but do we do it? Most of us don't. Patients often tell me, "It's just been too cold to get out and walk lately." Have we gotten that lazy, that complacent? It certainly has opened my eyes to the fact that, for many of us, maybe we've lost resiliency with the accoutrements and comforts of modern society.

My father played football for the Green Bay Packers back in 1949, often playing in frigid Wisconsin weather on a frozen gridiron. If I whined about much when I was growing up, he had one thing to say: "Toughen up!"

That may seem like a harsh thing to say to a young man growing up, but guess what? I'm no worse for wear. My dad expected me to be resilient because he knew it was in my best interest and would benefit me throughout my life, and it has.

I want to remind you that you are stronger than may believe. The things that set the *pros* apart from the rest of us are often simply the decisions that they make and the commitment that they are going to rise above the crowd, in whatever endeavor that they happen to choose. The *pros* also follow commitment with daily actions that tend to ensure their success.

I had the incredible opportunity recently to observe and learn from someone that I feel truly exemplifies what I'm talking about and what it means, in my mind, to be a real *pro*, in the broadest sense of the word. It reaffirmed to me what true commitment, dedication and goal-oriented perseverance truly means. I had the chance to see Bo Eason, a former collegiate All-American and safety for the Houston Oilers (from 1984-89), perform his semi-autobiographical play, *Runt of the Litter*, as well as hear him speak about the path that brought him to where he is today.

Bo grew up often being told he was too small to play football, an opinion which only served to fuel his fire. At the age of nine years old, Bo made a decision. He was going to achieve something big, something most young boys would not really consider seriously at that age. Bo took a crayon and paper and began to draw up a 20 year plan, the culmination of which would result in him playing professional football in the NFL, despite his young age and small stature at the time, and becoming the best safety in the league.

After playing high school ball, the fact that he didn't receive a college football scholarship didn't stop him from trying out for a small Division II college football team. However, he was sent home after only two days of practice, the coach informing him that he was just too small to play the game. But instead of going home, Bo went to the store and bought a loaf of bread and some peanut butter and slept in his car. You see, going home was never part of his plan. The following day, Bo simply showed back up to practice as if nothing had happened. The team trainers, knowing that he was not truly on the team at that point, relented in giving him a ragtag, ill-fitting helmet and practice uniform and Bo just kept showing up, day after day. His plan and the fact that quitting was not an option for him eventually paid off and earned him a spot on the team.

In 1984, Bo was the first safety chosen in the NFL draft. He played in the NFL for the next five years until his career was cut short due to repetitive knee injuries which required no less than seven surgeries during his football career.

Now, for someone who dedicated everything in his being, to becoming the very best football player that he could possibly be, playing at the highest level of the game, defying the odds and critics along the way, do you think Bo Eason allowed retirement from pro football to end his career? Not a chance.

A longstanding interest in theater ultimately took him to New York, where he studied acting and eventually led him to Hollywood. Along the way, Bo penned and began performing *Runt of the Litter*, a one-man play based on his own life and chronicling the 20 year plan he had begun at the age of nine. *Runt* details his life and eventual entry into the NFL, as he prepares for the final hour and culmination of his 20 year plan, the ultimate sibling face-off, pitting brother against brother in a championship, high-stakes playoff game, the winner of which is slated for a spot in the Super Bowl. In reality, the game never occurred, though it could have. Bo's brother, Tony Eason was the quarterback of the New

England Patriots and Bo played safety for the Houston Oilers. The two teams were scheduled to meet in the playoffs in the late 80s, but the game was derailed by a players strike.

As an off-Broadway play and up to the time of my own fortunate viewing of his performance, Bo has performed *Runt of the Litter* over 1200 times during the past decade, to critical acclaim and to audiences all across the country. The play has been bought by Frank Darabont (writer and director of *The Shawshank Redemption* and *The Green Mile*), with plans for adaptation to the screen.

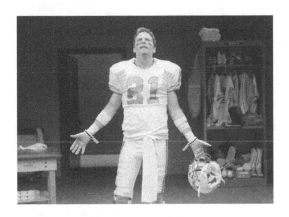

Bo Eason in his one-man hit play, **Runt of the Litter**

Bo was gracious enough to answer some questions from me, as I was especially curious about how he prepares himself routinely to perform *Runt of the Litter*, how he cares for himself, stays in shape and plans for the future. Here is what he had to say:

"When I'm doing the show (*Runt of the Litter*), my whole day is predicated on performing that show. I really have to eat well leading up to the show. What I eat and the timing of what I eat is very important, as I have performed this play for so long, I'm really conscious of what my body needs, and when, if I am to perform at my best. I am sometimes doing seven performances in a week and sometimes two in one day. If my nutrition is off, I really know it." The food; I am always thinking about it and I'm very in tune with how it affects my performance, both on stage and in my training."

"I can tell during a show if I haven't eaten well over the 12 hours preceding the play. I know what my body needs. The warm-up for the show is very physical, so I'll do a lot of stretching and plyometrics before a performance. I will typically lose 8-10 pounds of body-weight during the show, which I get back with re-hydration after the show and I'll follow the performance with a recovery shake which contains protein and all the electrolytes I need."

"When I'm on the road with the play, I will get up and do something every morning, whether it's just getting on the treadmill or doing something to get my body moving. I also work-out three mornings during the week, with a trainer, when I'm home and off the road. This takes place at a facility that caters to current and X-professional athletes or high caliber college athletes training for various sports, but it is a serious training facility with some of the best sports-specific trainers in the business. The caliber of the group that I work-out with is pretty high."

"The key for me is to work-out strenuously enough that it requires something of me. That always rights the ship for me. I've noticed that anytime my training slacks off, I may start to eat really crappy, and when my training is on track, my eating is on track, as well. So if I'm training consistently, my training always rights the ship, where my eating is concerned."

"I've always been very aware of nutrition and how to eat well, though that doesn't mean that I don't ever eat food, such as pizza, or have a beer on occasion. On the other-hand, I can also plan for things like that. Like if my wife and I want to go out for Mexican food and margaritas, I will plan for that and I don't beat myself up over that kind of stuff, because it's actually fun for me."

"I also know that if I have a few beers or a couple glasses of wine on a given night, I may feel it tomorrow and not perform the way I'd like the following day, so although I will occasionally have a planned night where I eat like this, I never make a habit out of doing those things on a more regular basis."

Dr. Kelley: "In watching your performance in *Runt of the Litter*, it is apparent that you deliver so much of yourself and it's such a physical performance. Do you have a long-term vision or view of how you plan to approach the future, as you get older, from the standpoint of your health and overall fitness?"

Bo: "Yeah, I actually was on an airplane recently; I'll be 50 this year and I just wrote this down in my 20 year plan. I decided that I want to get into the best shape that I possibly can be in over this next decade, between the age of 50 and 60. Not that I think I'll be able to do everything I could do when I was playing football, but I've got young kids and I want to continue to do all the things that dads do, such as have the ability to move and be active with them as they are involved in sports and other activities. My doctor, whom I've had for a long time, says my heart is like that of a 25 year old. He has joked and said, "Just promise me you won't get a beer belly, if you don't do that, you'll be fine."

"I've noticed that people who are high achievers or at least those who are considering the thought of being a high achiever, are never fat. They are almost always lean and they are very structured about how they eat and how they hydrate. That's part of their mechanism. Think about it; if you are not thinking about achieving something high, something significant, you don't necessarily have to ask that much from your body and your nutrition can be crappy. High achievers don't think like that, they are always thinking about how to fuel their bodies and very structured about how they go about doing that."

True professionals don't sit around waiting for their circumstances to change. They make things happen. They are often living examples of taking intangible thoughts, dreams and desires, and manifesting them into the reality they wish to create. The pros also expect a lot of themselves and they hold themselves accountable for creating much of their own success, including the way they take care of themselves.

I am going to challenge you to expect more from yourself, as well. Taking care of yourself through optimal diet and *daily* exercise is important. I am not going to lie to you and tell you it might not be demanding at times. However, as you develop the habit of doing so, you will change your life and have an impact on your health for the positive and possibly, forever.

There will always be naysayers around who somehow manage to disparage, criticize, and downplay the accomplishments of those who strive to achieve great things, even if those endeavors are focused solely on improving one's physical health and physical body. There will always be those who insist something is either not possible or not worth striving for. The pros, however, leave nothing to chance. They look at the goal or proposition ahead of them and set about the daily tasks which lead up to their desired outcome. I don't believe there is a better example of this than Bo Eason.

His brand has become a symbol which is synonymous with strength, endurance, perseverance and the ability to succeed, thrive and overcome adversity. As an actor, speaker and motivator, Bo has taken a seed which was planted as a nine year old boy with a dream and manifested that dream well beyond anything that most of us could have imagined.

Likewise, you too have the ability to decide that you are going to live an exceptional life. The pros don't put off what they have to do each day to improve and grow, no matter what their sport or business may be. Consequently, I am going to encourage you to begin to do the things that you know you need to do everyday, to succeed and to change your body, your health, and your life. You don't leave the house each day without brushing your teeth or taking a bath or shower. Getting in your exercise should be no different.

When I tell my patients to exercise *daily*, what I am really saying is to make it a priority and schedule it. Do you have to be perfect? No. Am I perfect? No, I am not. But I know this: If you don't plan to exercise each and every day and eat in a manner which supports your efforts, the less likely it is that those things will be accomplished. Do I ever miss a day of exercise? Of course I do and you will too, even if you commit to making fitness a way of life.

The difference is that by making the decision to bridge the gap between a more casual and occasional approach to your health and fitness, doing so will become habit sooner than you may think. You will likely reach a point where it is hard to imagine your life without this kind of daily routine.

Where your fitness and diet are concerned, I encourage you to **act like a pro**. Don't leave anything to chance. Make transforming your body to be the best it can be, a supreme priority in your life. Even if you have no ambition to become a competitive athlete or a bodybuilder, if you will commit to making your health a day-to-day priority, you won't believe how many other things in your life may improve, get easier or open up to you in the form of opportunity.

Fitness is one of those gifts that transcends itself. Fitness gives and gives and gives on so many levels. For the most part, it is free to all of us. I encourage you to reach for it and grab it! Don't wait another day to create a plan to get started on the road to taking care of you. I promise it will be worth your time, effort and commitment.

Chapter 18

Accountability Counts

Every new patient that I see at my clinic gets an Accountability Chart. An Accountability Chart is a simple, but very visual means of tracking your exercise progress and holding yourself accountable for getting out there (the gym, walking trail, etc.) and exercising.

I encourage my patients to place the Accountability Chart on a door, wall, the refrigerator, or any place that it will be unavoidable at some point in the day. Ideally, it acts as a reminder to them that there is something they need to take care of and accomplish for each day.

The Accountability Chart is simple to use and requires only that you place a checkmark or an X in each day's box, to signify and document that you have either completed or missed your exercise. I encourage far more checks to be placed than Xs.

But regardless of whether you use a chart or other means to document your exercise, having some means of holding yourself accountable to daily exercise can be a powerful motivator for staying on track.

One of the things many of my patients find most valuable about coming to our clinic is simply that we encourage them to come in weekly to weigh-in. This is not a mandatory requirement by any means. However, there is a clear correlation between patient progression in the weight-loss process when they hold themselves accountable to weigh-in each week.

I generally see steady, documented weight-loss progression over time with our patients who hold themselves accountable and allow us to hold them accountable week after week on their weight-loss journey. I cannot say the same for those patients whom I see less frequently. In fact, patients who choose not to come in for weekly weigh-ins seem to frequently struggle and often complain that they can't figure out why they're not progressing.

Take home message: Accountability counts. Find some manner to **hold yourself accountable** to staying on purpose. No one else can do this for you, though you can and should employ simple tools such as an Accountability Chart, as well as finding supportive friends, family or co-workers to help remind you daily, that you are on a mission and a journey to get healthier and to get fit.

Chapter 19

Track Your Progress (Journaling)

One other item we give to all of our new patients is a journal. The journal can be used in a variety of ways, but most importantly, we encourage people to write down or '**journal**' everything they put into their mouths day after day.

If you are trying to lose weight, it is very important to have a reasonable idea of the number and types (protein, fat, carbohydrate) of calories you are consuming each day.

It is well-known in the weight management field that diligent journaling correlates well with success. We have an innate tendency towards food amnesia, and many, many of us cannot remember what we had for lunch two days ago or yesterday, for that matter.

Journaling both your food intake as well as your daily exercise accomplishes a few things. First, it creates a record of your journey as you progress physically from point A to point B. Secondly; journaling creates a sense of mindfulness. As you journal your daily food intake, you become more mindful of everything you are putting in your mouth.

Increased mindfulness is important where food is concerned and from a practical standpoint, after you have put in 30 minutes or more of hard training, keeping **The Fitness Response** in mind, it becomes much less congruent to mindlessly devour a glazed donut at the office or eat in a random manner.

Journaling, when done with positive intent and used as a tool to help you stay on course, will provide the navigation points and blueprint that you can use to replicate your success, if you ever fall off course and regain some of the weight that you've lost.

Another form of journaling your progress and one that I strongly recommend is to track your progress through photographs. There really is nothing that more truthfully shows you where you are beginning, than by taking "before" pictures of your physique. You can have one or more views, taken in an outfit that doesn't leave much hidden. Taking a hard, honest look at your body in pictures can be both eye opening and motivating. You may find that you don't have as much of a journey as you thought. On the other hand, you may find that you have a worthwhile and important challenge to undertake.

By contrast, take an "after" picture at multiple points along your journey. You may want to document your progression every two weeks or once a month in photographic form. You can make these photographic documents as simple front and back views, or as detailed (front, back, side, arms, legs, etc.) as you wish.

Journaling is very personal for most people and a great source of self-accountability. If you are working with a trainer, nutritionist, physician, or coach, your journals, both written and photographic, can be used to help analyze your progress, help you and your mentor plan strategy and collaborate on your long-term goals.

Regardless of your ultimate intent in journaling, I encourage you to do it. Plan out and **journal, recording both your food and daily exercise.** In doing so, you create one more level of commitment to yourself and reinforce both behavior and lifestyle change in a big way that will pay off for years to come.

Chapter 20

Sleep like a Baby

Another complaint that I commonly hear is this: "Doc, I don't have any energy. What can I do to get more energy?" Low energy level can be the result of many different health-related issues and disorders, and if you are dealing with low energy, the first thing I'm going to encourage you to do is to see your physician about the issue.

However, in my own patient population, I will typically ask about these three things:

1. "Are you eating as well as you can eat?"
2. "Are you exercising everyday?"
3. "Are you getting enough sleep each night?"

If a patient's lab work is not troubling, I often find that one or more of these parameters are out of sync when someone is complaining about a lack of energy.

Lack of sleep is of particular concern because many of us are busier than ever. According to the National Sleep Foundation, there is no magic number of hours of sleep that applies to all of us. On the other hand, if you consistently stay up close to or beyond midnight and wake feeling less than well-rested or exhausted, you may need to reconsider if you're getting enough sleep.

From a muscle growth and recovery standpoint, it is well-known that inadequate sleep can result in decreased levels of testosterone and growth hormone (natural anabolic hormones), as well as increased levels of hormones such as cortisol which are catabolic in nature and lead to muscle breakdown and increased abdominal fat.

Inadequate sleep is a major culprit when it comes to optimal energy level. If you are exercising regularly, this alone will increase the probability that you will sleep better. The higher quality your nutrition, the more likely you will feel and function better every waking day. By the same token, lack of sleep can derail the best laid plans when it comes to not only your energy level, but to your physique development or transformation goals, as well.

On some level, this is common sense, but I also find that my patients who burn the midnight oil and stay up all hours of the night have more tendencies to drink alcohol and snack on high carbohydrate sources of junk food at the worst strategic time to be doing this.

If you are serious about improving your health and your body, **get a good night's sleep** every night, if at all possible. Tip the scales in the direction to give your body every advantage to grow, recover and optimize your muscle and body tissues. This is one case where the phrase "you snooze, you lose" just does not apply. Encourage your body to heal and recover. In doing so, you will affect your physical body and mental state in a very positive way, and in the process, you may very likely improve your energy level, as well!

Chapter 21

Become a Lifer

In January 2007, a cold-front blew in across Texas. I was still doing some emergency room work, but mostly only at night. On January 16, the roads in Austin had iced over. It made driving rather treacherous, considering that these freezes are fairly infrequent in this area.

For whatever reason, knowing that I was scheduled to work the night of January 17 and was off work during the day, I chose to stay around the house and didn't venture outside, instead choosing to lounge around, in anticipation of that night's ER shift.

Later in the afternoon, I noted that the sun had come out and it seemed to have warmed quite a bit. By the time I left for the hospital around 6 p.m., the roads appeared completely free of ice, that is, until I got to the highway.

I entered the on-ramp heading west on Highway 290. Only then did I see any signs of residual ice along the edges of the roadway. Still, I thought very little about it. By the time that I hit the first overpass, I was driving at a highway speed of 65 mph. Having been lulled into complacency by the otherwise clear roadways up until that point, it wasn't until I reached the edge of the overpass that I suddenly knew that I was in big trouble.

In an instant, I realized that I had absolutely no control over my 1999 Toyota 4-runner, as the backend began to fishtail wildly. Within seconds of entering the onramp, I was in a full-on, 360 degree spin, making several revolutions before finally slamming full speed into the concrete side retaining wall of the highway.

Fortunately for me, the driver side airbag deployed. Despite this, I walked away with a fractured sternum. This was my only injury, however, and I was grateful. I was 45 years old at the time and up until that particular day, on some level I had always felt some crazy sense of invulnerability. As I have alluded to earlier in the book, I have always maintained an active exercise schedule and felt I was in reasonably good shape at the time of the accident.

However, the days and weeks that followed informed me that I was not Superman. For the first time in my life and for several months thereafter, I felt like an old man. It seemed that every bone in my body ached. I struggled to pick up my then-three-year-old son, and getting down on the floor to play with him was out of the question.

I felt completely drained of energy and truly felt that I was in some sort of decline, from which I might not regain any sense of vibrancy or wellbeing. Gratefully, this was not the case. I slowly began to resume my regular exercise schedule and gradually got stronger. In the process, I began to notice that my joints became looser and I was beginning to move easier. Over the next several months, most of the pain I was having dissipated as my sternum healed and my energy level returned to that prior to the accident.

I tell you this story for a couple of reasons. First of all my accident made me acutely aware that we are more vulnerable to the unexpected than we consciously realize and bad things can happen to any of us, at any time. Secondly, however, we are also more resilient than we may believe, and how we respond to any challenge or adversity often comes down to the choices that we make in light of bad event.

Struggling with excess weight, for some of you, may be that adversity for which you see no real solution. You may have spent countless days, weeks, months, and even years trying to diet your weight away, all to no avail. You may feel hopeless and powerless because of this. If this is the case, then I truly feel for what you have struggled through. However, I also want to be completely candid with you.

Getting to where you truly want to go, physically speaking may not be as simple as decreasing your calories. Collectively, it seems we have a cultural belief that some new diet is going to be the one that makes all the weight go away. It will likely never be as simple a solution as that.

My entire purpose in writing this book has been to make it clear to you that in my experience and in my opinion, those who achieve consistent results in managing, transforming, and optimizing their physical body and their weight are generally doing *much more* than the average dieter, to make those results a reality. For those who maintain a high level of fitness, there is usually no mystery involved, and it is generally not by accident.

By all accounts, we are living much longer than previous generations. Financial experts are recommending against the traditional retirement at age 65 because many of us could possibly outlive any financial nest egg that we may have accumulated.

Point being, that one way or another, you may live much longer than you ever thought possible. If you want to increase the odds that you enter your later years in great health and with strength and vibrancy, I encourage you to consider taking a different tack. If you are fortunate enough to grow old and those years are truly to be "golden" years, then I suspect if, given the choice, you would want to enter them standing on your own two feet and on your own terms.

As you well know, not everyone ages the same or has the same good fortune of remaining mobile and active into and throughout their later years. For some, the sad reality will be the loss of independence and a loss of mobility. With a loss of mobility often comes a decline in general health, mental acuity, and the capacity to truly enjoy being alive.

It is my hope that you will make the decision to get yourself in shape and make doing so a priority. Decide that you are not only going to lose weight, but you are going to become stronger, and that you are going to make doing so, a daily priority. It is neither my purpose nor my desire to encourage you to become a bodybuilder or a competitive fitness athlete. I do, however, want to encourage you to make maintaining the strength and integrity of your body something that is a lifetime mission.

We have but one shot at this life and there are no guarantees. There is no guarantee that if you live a life striving for optimal health and fitness, you won't get cancer or get hit by a bus while crossing the street. We just don't know what is in store for us. However, I can tell you that as a physician who has cared for literally hundreds and thousands of patients over the course of my career, I have seen what the aftermath of neglect, complacency, and shear abuse of one's health can look like, and it is not pretty.

I have seen lifelong smokers in the end stages of chronic lung disease, gasping for breath like guppies out of water. I have seen methamphetamine addicts who have used up almost every available vein, consequently making the establishment of an intravenous line nearly impossible at a time when they truly required one for care.

I have seen and cared for many heart attack victims who may have thought that despite their poor diet, excess weight, and smoking habit, they would somehow be able to beat the odds.

I have watched as an obese patient, who should not have died, met her demise simply because her extreme excess weight precluded the establishment of an intravenous line by a team of highly experience healthcare workers.

I have seen many, many bad things happen to good people who just did not take care of themselves or abused their bodies with food, alcohol, tobacco, or drugs.

By contrast, because you have taken the time and made the choice to read this book, you have an opportunity to make an enormous positive change in your life. You can choose each and every day to live in a manner that may dramatically increase your odds of living a longer, healthier life.

As I said, there are no guarantees, but you have more control over your health than you think. In truth, you have more control over your health than does your doctor or anyone else, because you control every aspect of your ability to decide how you'll live your life, day to day.

I am going to encourage you to **become a lifer** and make the pursuit of optimal health, fitness, and nutrition a daily goal in your life. My hope is that you develop the daily habits that enable you to manage your weight and maintain your desired physique indefinitely.

By making your health and fitness your top priority, you will not be taking away from any other person or priority in your life. The only way you can truly care for your children, your family, or others in your life is to have first taken care of yourself.

On an airplane, we are always instructed to place the oxygen mask on ourselves first and then to take care of small children, in the event of loss of cabin pressure. As much as I hope none of us ever has to deal with that issue, it is a reminder that if we are to care for those around us, we must first be in a good condition ourselves.

Begin to take the best care of you that you possibly can. **Become a lifer**, and don't waiver in your commitment to a life of uncompromising health and fitness. I don't believe you will ever regret making this decision and sticking with it.

I wish you all the best as you pursue a path so few choose to follow.

Acknowledgments

This book would not have been possible without the help, input and advice of so many people. Most notably, however, I want to thank my wife Sherrill and my son Jake for their understanding and patience, while I spent countless hours hovering over the computer to complete this project. Thank you, Sherrill for your wisdom, input and perspective concerning this project.

I would like to thank David Sauer and Cindy Sauer for their initial time and effort in helping me to get my manuscript reviewed by Morgan-James Publishing. I would like to thank David Hancock, Rick Frishman and Jim Howard for their encouragement and enthusiastic support regarding the vision for the book.

I am also thankful for Stefanie Hartman and Tania Hartman, with SHE Inc., whose ongoing help and guidance have been so beneficial in helping me develop a means to spread my message in greater way, and for the opportunity to publish my book through Morgan-James Publishing and SHE Inc.

At Morgan-James Publishing, I'd like to especially thank my Author Relations Manager, Margo Toulouse, for her accessibility, expertise and guidance through the publishing process. I would also like to thank my PR and Marketing Liason, Bethany Marshall for all of her help, as well.

At Bomely Creative, I would like to thank Chris Bomely for his exceptional ability to bring visual form to life in a way that few people can and for his input and assistance at so many stages of this project, as well as so many others along the way.

I am especially appreciative of Bo Eason for both his time and generosity in contributing to the book and for fulfilling something in a big way that he teaches and speaks about; sharing oneself in a more generous way. Thank you, Bo. I also want to thank Dawn Eason, for her time, accessibility and for making possible my interview with Bo, as well as for providing a photograph from *Runt of the Litter*.

My gratitude goes out to Pattie Farley and Amalia Litras for everything that they have done in the way of allowing me to capture the true essence of what it means to <u>Live</u> The Fitness Response. Thank you both for your time and generosity. I wish you continued success. I would also like to thank Brook Jones for allowing us access to Hyde Park Gym for photography purposes.

Thank you to Madeleine Dimond at *Mousework Specialists* for her thoughtful editing of the book. as well as Tahila Mintz for her contributing photography. Thanks to Neysha Batchelor for her support in helping our patients implement The Fitness Response on a daily basis, and for everything she does to ensure that our clinic runs smoothly.

Last, but certainly not least, I want to thank Jack Lalanne, who sadly we lost this year. Thank you for showing us the path to follow and then leading the way like nobody else could. Your example was and continues to be, a fine example indeed. God bless you.

For more of Dr. Kelley's health, nutrition and fitness related information, please visit **RichardKelleyMD.com**

Additional Links

BoEason.com
This is the official website for Bo Eason, NFL Athlete, Screenwriter, Actor, Playwright and Speaker.

BomelyCreative.com
Bomely Creative is the collective design work of Chris Bomely. A full-service design studio based in Austin, Texas, Specializing in branding strategy and logo development.

GaryTaubes.com
Gary Taubes is an American science writer and the author of Nobel Dreams, Bad Science: The Short Life and Weird Times of Cold Fusion, Good Calories, Bad Calories and most recently, Why We Get Fat, And What to Do About It.

GrassIron.com
These Austin based fitness trainers have been helping everyday people achieve extraordinary results in weightlifting, power-lifting, bodybuilding, running and cycling. GrassIron is owned and operated by Amalia Litras and Pattie Farley.

HydeParkGym.com
An iconic fitness landmark in Austin and home to some of the best trainers in the area; this is the place where serious athletes and fitness enthusiasts go to train and stay fit.

JackLalanne.com
This is the official website of the late Jack Lalanne, father of the modern day fitness and health movement. This is the man that started it all!

PhysiciansWay.com
Physician's Way LLC is owned and operated by Richard and Sherrill Kelley. Physician's Way promotes healthy weight-management through the teaching of fitness-based lifestyle and nutrition strategies.

RuntOfTheLitter.com
Bo Eason's Semiautobiographical play, *Runt of the Litter*.

"One of the most powerful plays in the last decade" —*The New York Times*. You've got to see it!

ShireemImaging.com
ShireemImaging is the website of Tahila Mintz, documentary photographer, videographer and consultant.

To Learn More About
Dr. Kelley's Programs

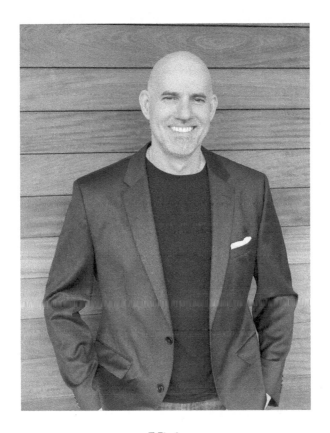

Visit

RichardKelleyMD.com

For a Ketogenic Approach to
The Fitness Response...

7 Day Keto Meal Plan

For

WEIGHT LOSS

A Guide to Intuitive Ketogenic Nutrition

Richard Kelley, M.D.

Join My Facebook Group and Download
Your **FREE** Guide
to Intuitive Ketogenic Nutrition
At

type2tohealth.com/ketuitivity